Emergency Management Anesthesia *and* Critical Care

Jeremy S. Heiner, EdD, CRNA, FAANA
Academic & Clinical Faculty
Kaiser Permanente School of Anesthesia
California State University, Fullerton
Pasadena, CA
USA

Mark Gabot, DNP, CRNA, FAANA
Academic & Clinical Faculty
Kaiser Permanente School of Anesthesia
California State University, Fullerton
Pasadena, CA
USA

Sass Elisha, EdD, CRNA, FAANA, FAAN
Assistant Director
Kaiser Permanente School of Anesthesia
California State University, Fullerton
Pasadena, CA
USA

ELSEVIER

Elsevier
3251 Riverport Lane
St. Louis, Missouri 63043

EMERGENCY MANAGEMENT IN ANESTHESIA   ISBN: 978-0-443-10693-4
AND CRITICAL CARE

Notice

Practitioners and researchers must always rely on their own experience and
knowledge in evaluating and using any information, methods, compounds or
experiments described herein. Because of rapid advances in the medical
sciences, in particular, independent verification of diagnoses and drug
dosages should be made. To the fullest extent of the law, no responsibility is
assumed by Elsevier, authors, editors or contributors for any injury and/or
damage to persons or property as a matter of products liability, negligence or
otherwise, or from any use or operation of any methods, products,
instructions, or ideas contained in the material herein.

Executive Content Strategist: Sonya Seigafuse
Senior Content Development Strategist: Vaishali Singh
Publishing Services Manager: Deepthi Unni
Project Manager: Sheik Mohideen K
Design Direction: Bridget Hoette

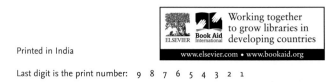

Working together
to grow libraries in
developing countries

www.elsevier.com • www.bookaid.org

Printed in India

Last digit is the print number: 9   8   7   6   5   4   3   2   1

We dedicate this book to all of the practitioners and students who provide high quality patient care every day. Furthermore, we hope that this information helps our educators guide the next generation of anesthesia and critical care professionals.

Preface

This book was written for academicians, clinicians, and students who are on the front lines caring for patients and managing emergencies every day. Additionally, this information will help educators design, conduct, and debrief critical event learning scenarios. Our intention is to help others continuously learn, improve, and perfect anesthesia and critical care practice. The information contained within these pages will expand the reader's knowledge related to diagnosing and treating crisis events that occur during anesthesia and critical care management.

This book is designed to "ride along" with the anesthesia and critical care professional in a scrub pocket or lab coat, so that it can be immediately available during an emergency. The emergency management topics are presented concisely, providing readers with all the necessary information in one resource. Each chapter begins with up-to-date management techniques for common and uncommon emergencies. We are confident that the information presented in this book will help to improve patient care.

Contents

SECTION 10   Obstetric Emergencies

SECTION 11   Equipment Emergencies

SECTION 12   Miscellaneous Emergencies

CHAPTER 1   Airway and Surgical Fire

MANAGEMENT

PRIMARY ACTIONS FOR AIRWAY FIRE

- Call for help
- Disconnect breathing circuit from the anesthesia machine
- Stop oxygen flow and ventilation
- Extinguish airway fire with sterile saline or water
- Remove tracheal tube and anything else in the airway (e.g., surgical sponges, temperature monitoring probe, etc.)
- Suction debris and fluids (e.g., segments of the burned endotracheal tube [ETT], and/or other debris that may remain in the airway)
- Reestablish a patent airway and resume ventilation/oxygenation
- Minimize FiO_2 by providing humidified O_2 to maintain a saturation of >90%
- Verify the extent of the injury using a flexible intubating (fiberoptic) endoscope
- Consider IV/inhaled corticosteroids and inhaled racemic epinephrine
- Consult burn specialists for advanced treatment
- Save all materials for investigation

PRIMARY ACTIONS FOR SURGICAL FIRE

- Call for help
- Disconnect breathing circuit from anesthesia machine
- Immediately remove burning drapes or other material from the patient
- Extinguish fire with CO_2 extinguisher, sterile saline, or water
- Activate the fire alarm/notify surgical team members
- Stop oxygen flow
- Manually ventilate with bag valve device
- Verify that the fire is extinguished
- Remove the patient from the operating room and close doors
- Turn off the gas supply to operating room (OR) suite
- Administer total IV anesthesia (if necessary) until the surgery can be completed
- Report all fires that occur within the OR to the hospital's risk management department

PREVENTION OF AIRWAY AND SURGICAL FIRES

- Conduct a fire risk assessment before every surgery and discuss fire prevention strategies

- Avoid open administration of supplemental O_2 and discontinue O_2 at least one minute before and during use of an ignition source (e.g., electrocautery or laser)
- Use low FiO_2 (maintain air/oxygen blend with an $FiO_2 \leq 30\%$) and communicate FiO_2 changes
- Reduce gas flow rates
- Avoid nitrous oxide
- Use manufactured laser-resistant ETT
- Fill endotracheal tube cuff with normal saline and dye in order to visualize cuff rupture
- Cover facial hair or other body hair with water soluble gel
- Protect the patient's eyes with wet gauze and laser goggles
- Avoid pooling of surgical preparation solutions
- Surgeon should communicate use of laser or electrocautery and avoid placing them on patient or on surgical drapes
- Use vented and flame-retardant drapes
- Soak sterile towels with sterile saline or water and place around surgical area
- Avoid petroleum-based ointments in surgical area
- Consider active evacuation of surgical gas/smoke with suction
- Moisten sponges that are used near ignition sources and consider protecting ETT with wet gauze
- Allow sufficient time for flammable skin preparations to dry (e.g., 120-180 seconds)
- Have sterile saline or water available to extinguish fire if it occurs
- Have fire extinguishers immediately accessible

MEDICATIONS

- IV corticosteroids (hydrocortisone 100 mg IV or dexamethasone 8 mg IV)
- Inhaled bronchodilators (albuterol) every 4 hours prn
- Inhaled racemic epinephrine every 4 hours prn for stridor or retractions

PHYSIOLOGY AND PATHOPHYSIOLOGY

It is estimated that between 550 to 650 airway and surgical fires occur within the United States each year. This devastating complication endangers the lives of patients and surgical personnel alike. Because a fire can engulf the entire OR in seconds, it is imperative that all anesthesia providers take measures to either prevent or decrease the potential for a fire and have a definitive plan if one occurs.

The three ingredients necessary to ignite a fire are a fuel source, an oxidizer, and an ignition source. The potential for a surgical fire exists because: (1) oxygen and nitrous oxide oxidizers exist in

Table 1-1 Commonly used lasers within the operating room

LASER	APPLICATION (SURGICAL SPECIALTY)
CO_2	General surgery, orthopedics, gynecology, urology, otolaryngology, plastic surgery
Nd:YAG	Gastroenterology, pulmonology, urology, dermatology, ophthalmology
Ho:YAG	Orthopedics, urology
Diode	Dermatology, ophthalmology, otolaryngology, plastic surgery, pain management
Argon	Ophthalmology, otolaryngology, plastic surgery, dermatology, gynecology

higher concentrations during anesthesia; (2) multiple heat/ ignition sources are used within the operating room (e.g., electrocautery, lasers, numerous electrical devices, defibrillators); and (3) fuel sources are in contact with the patient and staff (e.g., alcohol skin preps, surgical towels, gauze and sponges, drapes, gowns, ETT, face mask, or nasal cannula). Additionally, when lasers are used for surgical procedures, the concentrated energy may be focused within the airway. The laser beam may inadvertently penetrate the ETT or ignite surgical drapes resulting in a fire. A list of commonly used lasers is included in Table 1-1.

During an airway fire, both the heat and fire can be directed into the lungs, trachea, and upper airway causing catastrophic tissue damage, airway edema, and even death. Specific surgical procedures such as tracheostomy and tracheoesophageal fistula repair can increase the risk of airway fire because of the use of electrocautery within and around the airway and trachea. Anaerobic organisms such as *bacteroids* and *pepto-streptococci,* and aerobic organisms such as *staphylococci* and *Pseudomonas* may be present in patients with lung infections. The gas produced and emitted by these bacteria may increase the possibility of airway fires. Taking precautions to prevent airway and surgical fires is vital to patient safety. It is essential for the entire surgical team to work cohesively, identify fire risk, and formulate a comprehensive plan to protect the patient and OR staff from a surgical fire if it occurs.

SIGNS AND SYMPTOMS

Respiratory

- Decreased SpO_2
- Evidence of charred or burned airway tissue

- Stridor
- Wheezing

Cardiovascular

- Dysrhythmia
- Hypertension
- Tachycardia

Other considerations

- Inability to sustain positive pressure ventilation
- Large cuff leak during manual ventilation
- Loss of end tidal CO_2 waveform
- Machine alarms "low tidal volume"
- Odor of burning drapes or gauze
- Odor of burning tissue
- Odor of inhalation agent
- Smoke and fire
- Spark and/or popping sound
- Visual identification of fire
- Visual identification by surgeon of spark, cuff rupture, or fire

DIFFERENTIAL DIAGNOSIS

Respiratory

- Bronchospasm
- Endotracheal cuff rupture
- Hypercarbia
- Hypoxia
- Inadvertent endotracheal tube removal
- Stridor

Cardiovascular

- Cardiac arrest
- Cardiac dysrhythmias

Other considerations

- Acidosis
- Circuit disconnect
- Machine failure

Suggested Readings

- Enkhbaatar P, Pruitt Jr BA, Suman O, et al. Pathophysiology, research challenges, and clinical management of smoke inhalation injury. *Lancet*. 2016;388(10052):1437-1446.
- Higgins Roche BT. Anesthesia and laser surgery. In: Elisha S, Heiner JS, Nagelhout JJ, eds. *Nurse Anesthesia*. 7th ed. St. Louis: Elsevier; 2023:1085-1091.
- Jones TS, Black IH, Robinson TN, et al. Operating room fires. *Anesthesiology*. 2019;130:492-501.

CHAPTER 2   Acute Gastric Regurgitation/Aspiration

MANAGEMENT

PRIMARY ACTIONS

- Call for help
- Turn patient's head to the side (left lateral decubitus position)
- Suction gastric contents from oropharynx
- Apply cricoid pressure to decrease additional gastric aspiration, but AVOID cricoid pressure during active vomiting
- Immediate intubation
- Suction trachea and bronchi via endotracheal tube before ventilation
- Positive pressure ventilation with 100% FiO_2

SECONDARY ACTIONS

- Supportive ventilation strategy
  - 6-8 mL/kg tidal volume
  - PEEP 5-10 cm/H_2O
  - Titrate FiO_2 to SpO_2 >90%, PaO_2 >60 mm Hg
- Obtain baseline chest X-ray and arterial blood gas
- Bronchoscopy for removal of aspirated solids causing obstruction

PREVENTION:

- Identify risk factors for gastric aspiration (see Table 2-1)
- Adherence to current American Society of Anesthesiologists NPO guidelines
- Delay diagnostic or non-emergency surgical procedures
- Assess gastric volume using point-of-care ultrasound of the gastric antrum
- Select an alternative to general anesthesia (e.g., regional, neuraxial, monitored anesthesia care-conscious sedation with local anesthesia)
- Rapid sequence induction with application of cricoid pressure
- Nasogastric (NG) tube placement and suctioning prior to induction of anesthesia
- NG tube placement and suctioning after induction of anesthesia, if gastric distention occurs
- If patient is to remain intubated, place endotracheal tube with subglottic suction capability and provide continuous or intermittent suction
- Oropharyngeal suctioning before extubation

MEDICATIONS

- Pharmacologic prevention:
  - Metoclopramide 10-20 mg IV 20-30 minutes before induction of anesthesia
  - Famotidine 20 mg IV 60-90 minutes before induction of anesthesia
  - Sodium citrate 15-30 mL PO 20-30 minutes before induction of anesthesia
- Broad-spectrum antibiotics for bacterial pneumonia
- IV antibiotics specific to infective pathogen once identified by blood cultures
- Vasopressor and/or inotropic support for hemodynamic compromise

PHYSIOLOGY AND PATHOPHYSIOLOGY

During an induction of anesthesia, the upper and lower esophageal sphincters relax. Gastric aspiration can occur if intragastric pressure exceeds lower esophageal barrier pressure, such as during high ventilating pressures, increases in gastric volume, or a bowel obstruction. Three separate aspiration syndromes can exist separately or together: (1) chemical aspiration pneumonitis (also known as Mendelson syndrome); (2) mechanical obstruction; and (3) bacterial infection (which can lead to aspiration pneumonia).

Acute gastric aspiration can occur at any time throughout the anesthetic course while a patient's laryngeal reflexes are obtunded or inhibited. Gastric aspiration can migrate into the lungs, causing chemical pneumonitis, which can cause damage

Table 2-1 Risk factors for acute gastric aspiration

PATIENT-BASED FACTORS	PATHOPHYSIOLOGIC FACTORS	SITUATIONAL FACTORS
Full stomach Obstetric patients Lower esophageal sphincter tone Obesity Nausea and vomiting	• Gastrointestinal obstruction • Ascites • Diabetic gastroparesis • Gastroesophageal reflux disease • Hiatal hernia • Peptic ulcer disease • Acute head injury • Seizures • Parkinson disease	• Emergency surgery • Prolonged difficult airway management • Traumatic injury requiring surgical intervention

and inflammation of the pulmonary tissue and/or aspiration pneumonia from bacteria colonization. Mechanical obstruction results when solid or liquid aspirate obstructs any portion of the bronchopulmonary tree.

Initial concerns after acute gastric aspiration focus on chemical aspiration pneumonitis. This pathophysiologic process can be divided into two phases: phase 1 (direct chemical injury) and phase 2 (inflammatory mediator release). If aspirate reaches the pulmonary acinus, then chemical pneumonitis can result in atelectasis and hypoxia because of alveolar capillary membrane edema and degeneration, alveolar type II pneumocyte destruction, and microhemorrhaging. Management of this condition frequently requires positive pressure ventilation and is mainly supportive.

The earliest and most reliable sign of acute gastric aspiration is hypoxia. The severity of the signs and symptoms are dependent on the:
1) volume aspirated
2) pH of the aspirate
3) type of aspirate (solids cause more pulmonary tissue damage that liquids)
4) patient's physical condition and comorbidities

SIGNS AND SYMPTOMS

Respiratory

- Chest X-ray infiltrates
- Dyspnea
- Gastric secretions in oropharynx
- Hypercarbia
- Hypoxemia (earliest and most reliable sign)
- Increased positive inspiratory pressure
- Rales/rhonchi
- Tachypnea
- Wheezing

Cardiovascular

- Initial hypertension followed by hypotension if aspiration is severe
- Pulmonary hypertension
- Tachycardia

Other considerations

- Disseminated intravascular coagulation

DIFFERENTIAL DIAGNOSIS

Respiratory

- Acute respiratory distress syndrome
- Bronchospasm
- Endotracheal tube migration/obstruction
- Hypercarbia
- Hypoxia
- Pneumonia
- Pulmonary edema
- Pulmonary embolism
- Upper respiratory tract infection

Cardiovascular

- Congestive heart failure

Other considerations

- Anaphylaxis

Diagnostic tests

- Chest X-ray
- Arterial blood gas
- Sputum cultures to identify pathogen

Suggested Readings

- Borshoff DC. *The Anaesthetic Crisis Manual*. International ed., Version 2. D.C. Borshoff; 2017.
- Heiner JS. Respiratory anatomy, physiology, pathophysiology, and anesthesia management. In: Elisha S, Heiner JS, Nagelhout JJ, eds. *Nurse Anesthesia*. 7th ed. St. Louis: Elsevier; 2023:614-679.
- Kollmeier BR, Keenaghan M. Aspiration risk. [Updated 2022 Jan 19]. In: *StatPearls* [Internet]. Treasure Island, FL: StatPearls Publishing; 2022. Available at: https://www.ncbi.nlm.nih.gov/books/NBK470169/.
- Raghavendran K, Nemzek J, Napolitano LM, Knight PR. Aspiration-induced lung injury. *Crit Care Med*. 2011;39(4):818-826.

CHAPTER 3 Emergent Reintubation

MANAGEMENT

PRIMARY ACTIONS

- Provide 100% FiO_2 and sit patient upright if possible
  - Verify SpO_2, $EtCO_2$, and blood pressure reading
- Call for help and a video laryngoscope
- Communicate with the team and create a rapid plan for oxygenation/reintubation
- Support ventilation with a bag-valve-mask or anesthesia breathing circuit and mask
- Perform a rapid sequence induction (RSI)
  - Reintubate with direct or video laryngoscopy and have suction readily available
- If contraindications to succinylcholine exist, consider:
  - Rocuronium (see "Medications")
  - Cisatracurium (see "Medications")
  - Reintubation without neuromuscular blocking agent
- Perform crash intubation with RSI if signs of cardiorespiratory decline
- Identify and manage primary cause of respiratory decompensation

SECONDARY ACTIONS

- Prior to extubation, perform an endotracheal tube (ETT) cuff leak test
- Always consider reintubation with a smaller size ETT
- Treat stridor with oxygen, racemic epinephrine, and corticosteroids if $SpO_2 > 90\%$ (see "Medications")
  - Reintubate with smaller size ETT if there are signs of respiratory decompensation

MEDICATIONS

- For RSI
  - Propofol 0.2-2 mg/kg IV or,
  - Ketamine 0.5-2 mg/kg IV
  - Succinylcholine 1-1.5 mg/kg IV
  - If contraindications to succinylcholine exist consider:
    - Rocuronium 1-1.2 mg/kg IV
      - If no recent neuromuscular-blocking reversal agent has been administered
    - Cisatracurium 0.15-0.3 mg/kg IV
      - If sugammadex was used for reversal of neuromuscular blockade
      - Not recommended for RSI due to onset of 2-3 minutes

- Postoperative stridor
  - Racemic epinephrine 0.5 mL of 2.25% solution diluted in 3 mL normal saline via nebulizer every 3-4 hours
  - Decadron 0.15 mg/kg IV or,
  - Hydrocortisone 100 mg IV or,
  - Methylprednisolone 20 mg IV
- Provide cardiovascular support to maintain mean arterial pressure > 65 mm Hg:
  - Ephedrine 5-10 mg IV bolus and/or,
  - Phenylephrine 50-100 mcg IV bolus, 0.1-0.5 mcg/kg/min infusion and/or,
  - Epinephrine 10-100 mcg IV bolus, 0.1-0.5 mcg/kg/min infusion and/or,
  - Norepinephrine 5-10 mcg IV bolus, 0.1-0.5 mcg/kg/min infusion

PHYSIOLOGY AND PATHOPHYSIOLOGY

Emergent reintubation is a critical event that can be associated with significant morbidity and mortality. It primarily occurs because of unexpected or failed tracheal extubation, respiratory decompensation, or cardiovascular compromise (see Table 3-1).

Table 3-1 Factors that increase the risk of emergent postoperative reintubation

Patient factors	• Age < 1 year and > 65 years • ASA physical status III or greater • Excessive airway secretions • Hemodynamic instability • Laryngospasm/bronchospasm • Phrenic nerve dysfunction • Preoperative anemia (hematocrit < 34%) • Preoperative hypoalbuminemia (albumin < 3.5 g/dL) • Short/thick neck • Tracheal pathology (tracheal stenosis or tracheo-malacia)
Comorbidities	• Chronic pulmonary disease (e.g., COPD) • Congestive heart failure • Pulmonary edema • Renal insufficiency (serum creatinine > 1.2 mg/dL or CrCl < 70 mL/min), especially if patient requires dialysis • Sepsis

Continued

Table 3-1 Factors that increase the risk of emergent postoperative reintubation—cont'd

Anesthetic factors	• Excessive fluid administration with resulting pulmonary edema • Inadequate reversal of neuromuscular blockade • Multiple, traumatic attempts at airway management and intubation • Overinflated ETT cuff • Oversized endotracheal tube causing vocal cord or tracheal swelling • Recent administration of excessive opioid or anesthetic agents • Vocal cord damage
Surgical factors	• Surgical time greater than 3 hours • Adverse reaction to blood products or medications • Head, neck, and thoracic surgery • Postsurgical bleeding (especially within the airway) • Surgical error • Vocal cord or recurrent laryngeal nerve damage
Types of cases	• Emergency surgery • Head and neck surgery • Cardiothoracic surgery • Airway surgery
Other factors	• Prolonged intubation (> 36 hours) • Recurrent intubations • Agitation while intubated

Abbreviations: ASA, American Society of Anesthesiologists; CrCl, creatine clearance; ETT, endotracheal tube.

A primary reason for emergent reintubation after anesthesia is due to residual neuromuscular blockade. This postanesthesia complication can be confirmed by assessing a train-of-four ratio less than 0.9, or clinical indications such as pharyngeal and upper airway muscle weakness, impaired swallowing, impaired chest excursion during spontaneous ventilation, and a generalized reduction in respiratory muscle tone. Complications associated with residual neuromuscular blockade include an increased risk of aspiration, upper airway obstruction, hypoxemia, and impaired oxygenation.

Administration of succinylcholine which is used for rapid neuromuscular blockade causing paralysis may be prolonged if an anticholinesterase (e.g., neostigmine) was used for reversal of neuromuscular blockade, especially in patients with chronic renal insufficiency.

However, succinylcholine administration after the use of sugamma-dex will not affect the onset or offset of paralysis.

Postoperative stridor is a concerning sign and represents potential airway compromise. Damage or swelling to the vocal cords or recurrent laryngeal nerve damage can occur from surgical intervention near these structures. Aggressive and/or prolonged airway management, an inappropriately sized ETT, and excessive ETT cuff inflation can occur in combination or separately, and may lead to both vocal cord damage and tracheal swelling causing postoperative stridor.

SIGNS AND SYMPTOMS

Neurologic
- Altered level of consciousness

Respiratory
- Decreased respiratory effort
- Hoarseness
- Stridor
- Subcutaneous emphysema
- Tracheal swelling
- Wheezing

Cardiovascular
- Dysrhythmia
- Hyper- or hypotension
- Signs of postoperative bleeding
- Tachycardia

Musculoskeletal
- Decreased neuromuscular stimulation (e.g., reduced train-of-four and tetanus during stimulation)
- Poor respiratory muscle effort (e.g., diaphragm and/or external intercostal muscle weakness)

Other considerations
- Known respiratory nerve or respiratory muscle damage
- Recent administration of opioids or anesthetic medications
- Residual neuromuscular blockade

DIFFERENTIAL DIAGNOSIS

Neurologic
- Acute cerebrovascular accident
- Neuroleptic malignant syndrome

- Postoperative cognitive dysfunction
- Recurrent laryngeal nerve damage
- Seizures

Respiratory

- Aspiration syndrome
- Upper or lower airway obstruction

Cardiovascular

- Myocardial infarction
- Postsurgical hemorrhage

Endocrine

- Addison disease
- Cushing disease
- Hypoparathyroidism
- Hypothyroidism

Pharmacologic

- Opioid administration
- Residual anesthesia
- Prolonged neuromuscular blockade
- Serotonin syndrome

Musculoskeletal

- Malignant hyperthermia

Other considerations

- Electrolyte abnormalities (e.g., calcium, sodium, potassium, and/or magnesium)

Diagnostic tests

- Obtain electrolytes, complete blood count, renal function tests, and serum albumin
- Head computed tomography scan
- Chest radiograph
- Electrocardiogram
- Cardiac markers (e.g., troponin level)

Suggested Readings

- Acheampong D, Guerrier S, Lavarias V, et al. Unplanned post-operative reintubation following general and vascular surgical procedures: outcomes and risk factors. *Ann Med Surg (Lond)*. 2018;33:40-43.
- Chen S, Zhang Y, Che L, Shen L, Huang Y. Risk factors for unplanned reintubation caused by acute airway compromise after general anesthesia: a case-control study. *BMC Anesthesiol*. 2021;21(1):17.
- Iwasaki H, Renew JR, Kunisawa T, et al. Preparing for the unexpected: special considerations and complications after sugammadex administration. *BMC Anesthesiol*. 2017;17(1):140.
- Siddiqui KM, Samad K, Jonejo F, Khan MF, Ahsan K. Factors affecting reintubations after cardiac and thoracic surgeries in cardiac intensive care unit of a tertiary care hospital. *Saudi J Anaesth*. 2018;12(2):256-260.
- Heiner JS. Respiratory anatomy, physiology, pathophysiology, and anesthesia management. In: Elisha S, Heiner JS, Nagelhout JJ, eds. *Nurse Anesthesia*. 7th ed. St. Louis: Elsevier; 2023: 614-679.

CHAPTER 4   Failed Airway

MANAGEMENT

PRIMARY ACTIONS

- Call for help
- Get difficult airway cart
- Increase FiO_2 to 100%
- Attempt face mask ventilation with two hands while assistant ventilates with anesthesia circuit and mask or bag-valve-mask
- If mask ventilation fails, attempt ventilation with supraglottic airway (SGA)
- Verify adequate ventilation with consistent $ETCO_2$ waveform capnography, bilateral chest rise, and equal and bilateral lung sounds

Ventilation inadequate

- Oxygenation is the highest priority — Continuously monitor time, patient $ETCO_2$, and patient SpO_2
- A brief attempt with a video laryngoscope is acceptable if direct laryngoscopy fails and SpO_2 is not critically low (e.g., $< 90\%$), or if intubation has not been attempted
- Confirm paralysis (see "Medications")
  - Consider one final attempt with face mask ventilation
- Prepare equipment for needle, wire-guided, or surgical cricothyrotomy
- Optimize position and identify the cricothyroid membrane (CTM)
- Sterilize the CTM with preparation solution (e.g., betadine or chlorhexadine)
- Place cricothyrotomy
- Confirm adequate ventilation with consistent $ETCO_2$ waveform capnography, bilateral chest rise, and equal and bilateral lung sounds
- Facilitate exhalation through upper airway with a jaw thrust, oral and/or nasal airway, or SGA

SECONDARY ACTIONS

Ventilation adequate

- Continuously monitor for adequacy of ventilation
- Consider awakening patient
- Remain mindful of time and limit intubation attempts to three or fewer
- Consider additional administration of a sedative hypnotic and a neuromuscular blocker (see "Medications")
- Use airway adjuncts for intubation and avoid blind intubation (see Table 4-1 for airway adjuncts)
- Options for intubation:
  - Intubation through existing SGA using flexible intubating bronchoscope
  - Video laryngoscopy in conjunction with bougie stylet

- Intubating SGA with ETT placement through intubating SGA using flexible intubating bronchoscope
- Combination of video laryngoscopy and flexible bronchoscopy — video laryngoscopy-inclusive flexible intubation (VIFI)
- Confirm ETT placement with consistent $ETCO_2$ waveform capnography, bilateral chest rise, and equal and bilateral lung sounds
- Report failed intubation and failed oxygenation in patient's medical record

MEDICATIONS

- Sedative hypnotics
  - Propofol 0.2-2 mg/kg IV or,
  - Ketamine 0.1-1 mg/kg IV
- Neuromuscular blocker
  - Succinylcholine 1.5-2 mg/kg IV or,
  - Rocuronium 1.0-1.2 mg/kg IV

Table 4-1 Difficult airway adjuncts

AIRWAY DEVICE	INDICATIONS
Standard laryngo-scope with multiple blades (straight, curved, Miller, MacIntosh, and Flex Tip blades)	• Difficult laryngoscopy and/or intubation • Difficult use of a supraglottic airway • Consider curved blade in the presence of a large tongue • Consider straight blade in the presence of an elongated epiglottis • Flex Tip blade bends 70° further depressing the hyoepiglottic ligament in the vallecula to provide additional lift to the epiglottis
Flexible intubating (fiberoptic) bronchoscope	• Anticipated difficult laryngoscopy and/or intubation • Awake ETT placement (consider antisiala-gogue, local anesthesia, and sedation) • Decreased cervical range of motion • Decreased thyromental and/or thyrohyoid distance (anterior larynx) • Mallampati class IV • Mandibular hypoplasia • Restricted mouth opening • Upper airway obstructions (tumors, pathology) • Visual confirmation of ETT placement • Use requires experience • Excessive blood and/or secretions can obstruct view

Continued

Table 4-1 Difficult airway adjuncts—cont'd

AIRWAY DEVICE	INDICATIONS
Video laryngoscope (e.g. Glidescope, McGrath, Karl Storz C-MAC)	• Anticipated/unanticipated difficult laryngoscopy and/or intubation • Awake or asleep ETT placement • Cormack-Lehane grade 3 or 4 • Decreased cervical range of motion • Decreased mouth opening • Decreased thyromental and/or thyrohyoid distance (anterior larynx) • Head, facial, and/or neck trauma • Mallampati class III or IV • Mandibular hypoplasia • Out of OR emergency airway management • Visual confirmation of ETT placement • Excessive blood and/or secretions can obstruct view
Supraglottic devices (e.g., LMA Classic, LMA Supreme, Ambu LMA, CobraPLA, PAXpress, Cookgas ILA)	• Can facilitate intubation when difficult laryngoscopy and/or intubation occurs • Rescue ventilation when mask ventilation is inadequate • Use flexible intubating (fiberoptic) bronchoscope through supraglottic device to visualize and verify ETT placement
Intubating supraglottic airway (LMA Fastrach, LMA C-Trach, Air-Q)	• Anticipated/unanticipated difficult laryngoscopy and/or intubation • Can facilitate intubation when difficult laryngoscopy and/or intubation occurs • Decreased cervical range of motion • Decreased thyromental and/or thyrohyoid distance (anterior larynx) • Head and facial trauma • Mandibular hypoplasia • Out of OR emergency airway management • Use flexible intubating (fiberoptic) bronchoscope through supraglottic device to visualize and verify ETT placement
Eschmann stylet (gum elastic bougie)	• Cormack-Lehane grade 2, 3, or 4 • Difficult intubation • Facilitates ETT delivery when using video laryngoscope • Requires minimal training

Table 4-1 Difficult airway adjuncts—cont'd

AIRWAY DEVICE	INDICATIONS
Lighted stylet (Laerdal Trachlight)	• Difficult airway • Not recommended by many difficult airway algorithms due to potential for trauma from blind intubation technique
Rigid and semi-rigid fiberoptic stylets (Shikani optical stylet, Levitan "First Pass Success" scope, Bonfils Retromolar Intubation Fiberscope, Rigid Intubating Fiber-optic Laryngoscope)	• Decreased cervical range of motion • Decreased thyromental and/or thyrohyoid distance (anterior larynx) • Difficult laryngoscopy and/or intubation • Restricted mouth opening • Excessive blood and/or secretions can obstruct view
Optically enhanced laryngoscopes (Airtraq)	• Decreased cervical range of motion • Difficult laryngoscopy and/or intubation • Decreased thyromental and/or thyrohyoid distance (anterior larynx) • Restricted mouth opening • Excessive blood and/or secretions can obstruct view
Esophageal tracheal tube (Combitube, King LT Airway, Rusch EasyTube)	• Difficult laryngoscopy and/or intubation • Difficult mask ventilation • Difficult placement of a supraglottic device • Use can be considered during preparation for a cricothyrotomy
Retrograde wire	• Not recommended due to blind technique
Cricothyrotomy (needle, wire-guided, or surgical)	• Emergency airway management (e.g., cricothyrotomy) • Cannot intubate, cannot oxygenate • Trauma to supralaryngeal structures • Intubation is contraindicated or deemed impossible

PHYSIOLOGY AND PATHOPHYSIOLOGY

A "failed airway" occurs when there is an inability to ventilate and oxygenate a patient with an obtunded airway. This can result from an anticipated or an unanticipated difficult airway. Indications, signs, symptoms, and considerations for patients at risk for a difficult airway are noted in Table 4-2.

One type of "failed airway" occurs when primary attempts at airway management are unsuccessful and alternative airway interventions are ineffective at maintaining oxygenation. A clinical example includes failure to intubate, with subsequent failed attempts using facemask ventilation and/or supraglottic airway ventilation. This is commonly termed the "cannot intubate, cannot oxygenate" scenario and is an emergency. It must be promptly

Table 4-2 Indications, signs, symptoms, and considerations for patients at risk for a difficult airway

ASSESSMENT	SIGNS AND/OR SYMPTOMS	CONSIDERATIONS
Difficult mask ventilation	• Beard • Edentulous • Redundant airway tissue • Mass on the face or neck • Decreased cervical range of motion • Wheezing • Stridor • Snoring • Altered mandibular or maxillary anatomy • Vomiting • Blood or excessive secretions in the airway • Foreign body in the airway • Increased peak inspiratory pressures (PIP) • Obesity • Pregnancy	• Enlarged upper and lower airway mass or a gravid uterus may cause altered ventilation by way of increased PIP's and increased pressure on the diaphragm (consider raising head of bed) • Use of muscle paralysis in the presence of an upper or lower airway mass may lead to an inability to ventilate/intubate (consider changing the patient position) • Increased PIP's resulting from foreign body, bronchospasm, ARDS, pulmonary infection, and/or pulmonary edema • Initial proper patient positioning can aid in effective mask ventilation • Consider muscle paralysis to facilitate ventilation in situations where a patient's muscular contraction may interfere with ventilation attempts

Table 4-2 Indications, signs, symptoms, and considerations for patients at risk for a difficult airway—cont'd

ASSESSMENT	SIGNS AND/OR SYMPTOMS	CONSIDERATIONS
Difficult laryngoscopy and/or intubation	• Altered airway anatomy • Mandibular hypoplasia • Large tongue • Short neck • Increased neck circumference greater than 43 cm at the level of the thyroid cartilage • Decreased cervical range of motion • Prominent incisors • Dental abnormalities (e.g., loose teeth) • Mouth opening < 3 finger breadths • Temporomandibular joint dysfunction • Thyromental distance < 3 finger breadths • Thyrohyoid distance < 2 finger breadths (e.g., anterior larynx) • Mallampati class III or IV • Poor view of the glottis (Cormack-Lehane grade 3 or 4) • Upper airway mass • Goiter • Vomiting • Blood or excessive secretions in the airway • Pregnancy • Obesity	• Scarring, masses, blood, vomit, excessive mucus, burns, or trauma could distort visualization during direct laryngoscopy or video laryngoscopy • Upper airway anatomy can be altered during pregnancy due to swelling of soft tissue • Muffled or hoarse voice, dysphagia, stridor, and/or dyspnea are indications of upper airway obstruction • Conservative administration of sedatives in the presence of an upper airway obstruction or identified difficult laryngoscopy to maintain respiration

Continued

Table 4-2 Indications, signs, symptoms, and considerations for patients at risk for a difficult airway—cont'd

ASSESSMENT	SIGNS AND/OR SYMPTOMS	CONSIDERATIONS
Difficult use or placement of a supra-glottic device	• Mouth opening < 3 finger breadths • Temporomandibular joint dysfunction • Prominent incisors • Dental abnormalities (e.g. loose teeth) • Airway obstruction above/below the larynx • Distorted airway anatomy • Angioedema • Decreased cervical range of motion • Increased peak in-spiratory pressures (PIP)	• Upper airway masses, swelling, foreign bodies, or redundant tissue may compromise the seal and ventilatory capability of the supraglottic device • Increased PIP may be a result of a foreign body, bronchospasm, ARDS, pulmonary infection, and/or pulmonary edema
Difficult crico-thyrotomy or surgical tra-cheotomy	• Scarring of the larynx or neck (e.g., surgery or radiation) • Neck hematoma or mass (e.g., abscess, tumor) • Short neck • Goiter • Obesity • Subcutaneous emphysema • Decreased cervical range of motion	• The location of a possible cricothyrotomy or trache-otomy should be identi-fied during the preopera-tive airway assessment • Cricothyrotomy is most often reserved for emer-gency situations • Equipment for cricothyrot-omy should be prepared before airway manipula-tion if there are indica-tions of potential failure with airway management • Consider muscle paralysis to facilitate cricothyrotomy

treated to avoid critical oxygen desaturation ($SpO_2 < 80\%$) and cerebral hypoxia.

Most difficult airway algorithms and failed airway checklists focus on limiting intubation attempts to three or fewer to prevent upper airway trauma, which may cause bleeding, edema, and the inability to ventilate. In addition, these sources recommend attempting ventilation quickly when primary intubation attempts are unsuccessful. An awareness of time and the adequacy of ventilation and oxygenation, by monitoring $ETCO_2$ waveform capnography and SpO_2, is essential. These airway resources promote communication with the airway team regarding unsuccessful attempts at airway management, and subsequent airway management strategies the operator plans to perform. Neuromuscular blockade is recommended after failed attempts at intubation and ventilation when awakening the patient is not an option. Neuromuscular blockade can help (1) improve the ability to ventilate, and (2) allow for optimal conditions if performing a cricothyrotomy.

If multiple airway management plans fail and hypoxemia is present with no detectible $ETCO_2$ (despite multiple attempts at ventilation), then cricothyrotomy is recommended. The three types of cricothyrotomy are needle, wire-guided, and surgical. A needle cricothyrotomy is a large-bore catheter transcutaneously placed through the CTM and used in combination with a transtracheal jet ventilator. A wire-guided cricothyrotomy uses a cricothyrotomy kit to place a larger bore catheter over a wire (e.g., Seldinger technique) through the CTM and into the trachea. An operator can then ventilate using a bag valve mask or anesthesia circuit and mask. The surgical technique for placing a cricothyrotomy uses a scalpel to cut through the CTM. A bougie stylet or tracheal forceps can then facilitate placement of a tracheal tube into the trachea.

Another type of "failed airway" occurs when initial intubation attempts have failed, but ventilation and oxygenation are successful. This is also known as the "cannot intubate, can oxygenate" scenario. In this situation, an airway operator has time to perform other airway interventions (see Table 4-1) or can elect to awaken the patient. Updated airway algorithms support the use of video-assisted intubation techniques and recommend avoiding blind intubation techniques. Vigilant monitoring of time and the adequacy of ventilation during airway management is vital.

SIGNS AND SYMPTOMS

Neurologic

• Loss of consciousness

Respiratory

• Absent $ETCO_2$ waveform
• Airway contamination (e.g., blood, vomit)
• Apnea
• Cyanosis and pallor
• Decreasing SpO_2
• Hypoxia
• Airway trauma

Cardiovascular

• Arrhythmias
• Cardiovascular collapse with severe hypoxemia
• Heart rate:
   - Early hypoxemia: tachycardia
   - Late hypoxemia: bradycardia
• Hypertension with hypoxemia

Other considerations

• Consider indications for a difficult airway (see Table 4-2)
• Failed face mask and SGA ventilation and oxygenation
• Two or more failed attempts at intubation

DIFFERENTIAL DIAGNOSIS

Respiratory

• Acute respiratory distress syndrome (ARDS)
• Airway obstruction (upper)
• Airway trauma
• Altered airway anatomy (e.g., tumors, goiters, scarring)
• Angioedema
• Bronchospasm (severe)
• Laryngospasm
• Ludwig angina
• Pneumothorax or tension pneumothorax
• Pulmonary edema
• Pulmonary embolus
• Smoke inhalation

Cardiovascular

• Myocardial infarction

Other considerations

- All shock states
- Mechanical: circuit/machine failure, pulse oximetry probe mal-position, or circuit or $ETCO_2$ line disconnect

Diagnostic Tests

- Ultrasound of the upper airway, larynx, and cricothyroid membrane
- Computed tomography or magnetic resonance imaging scans of the upper airway (when indicated for masses or other pathology)

Suggested Readings

- Apfelbaum JL, Hagberg CA, Connis RT, et al. 2022 American Society of Anesthesiologists Practice Guidelines for Management of the Difficult Airway. *Anesthesiology*. 2022;136:31-81.
- Ariadne Labs. *Ariadne Labs OR Crisis Checklists*. May 2017. Available at: https://www.ariadnelabs.org/resources/downloads/ariadne-labs-or-crisis-checklists-updated-2017/#. Accessed April 13, 2022.
- Frerk C, Mitchell VS, McNarry AF, et al. Difficult Airway Society intubation guidelines working group, Difficult Airway Society 2015 guidelines for management of unanticipated difficult intubation in adults. *Br J Anaesth*. 2015;115(6):827-848.
- Heiner JH. Airway management. In: Elisha S, Heiner JS, Nagelhout JJ, eds. *Nurse Anesthesia*. 7th ed. St. Louis: Elsevier; 2023:429-476.

CHAPTER 5 Laryngospasm

MANAGEMENT

PRIMARY ACTIONS

- Provide FiO_2 100%
- Confirm airway patency (e.g., place or reposition an oropharyngeal or nasopharyngeal airway)
- Perform a jaw thrust and apply pressure posterior to mandibular angle (laryngospasm notch)
- Manual ventilation with application of continuous positive airway pressure
- For persistent, inadequate ventilation and/or oxygenation, administer succinylcholine (see "Medications")

SECONDARY ACTIONS

- Monitor for signs and symptoms of negative pressure pulmonary edema
- Reintubation as necessary
- If ventilation remains inadequate after the administration of succinylcholine or nondepolarizing neuromuscular blockade, consider severe bronchospasm as the definitive cause

MEDICATIONS

- Succinylcholine adult dose 0.2-0.5 mg/kg IV (approximately 40 mg)
- Succinylcholine pediatric dose 2-3 mg/kg IV or 4-5 mg/kg IM; and administer atropine 0.01-0.02 mg/kg to prevent bradycardia
- If succinylcholine is contraindicated, administer rocuronium 1 mg/kg IV bolus

PHYSIOLOGY AND PATHOPHYSIOLOGY

Laryngospasm is a primitive, protective laryngeal reflex that occurs in response to various noxious stimuli in the airway (e.g., laryngeal mask airway, water, mucus, blood). The precise neural pathway and the mechanical mechanism by which laryngospasm occurs are not fully understood. However, laryngospasm is most likely caused by the combined contraction of multiple laryngeal muscles. One possible explanation for this physiologic reflex proposes that noxious stimuli transmit an afferent sensory response from the glottis to the internal branch of the superior laryngeal nerve. Subsequently, an efferent motor response via the external branch of the superior laryngeal nerve activates the cricothyroid muscles, stimulating them to contract, resulting in laryngospasm.

A laryngospasm can result in partial or full closure of the vocal cords. A partial laryngospasm can result in a high-pitched "crowing" sound, which is associated with a decreased ability to provide adequate tidal volume during ventilation with a mask or supraglottic airway device. Successful treatment of a partial laryngospasm can be achieved by rapidly increasing the depth of anesthesia and/or providing continuous positive airway pressure.

SIGNS AND SYMPTOMS

Respiratory

- Abnormal or absent $EtCO_2$ waveform
- Cyanosis
- Desaturation
- Hypercarbia
- Hypoxemia
- Inadequate face mask ventilation
- Inspiratory or expiratory stridor (e.g., partial laryngospasm)
- Intercostal and/or suprasternal inspiratory retractions
- Increased peak pressure
- Negative pressure pulmonary edema
    1. Bilateral rales
    2. Desaturation
    3. Pink frothy or exudative pulmonary secretions
    4. Radiographic evidence of pulmonary edema
- Oral secretions/blood
- Paradoxical chest and abdominal movement (rocking or seesaw)
- Tracheal tugging on inspiration

Cardiovascular

- Bradycardia (late sign of hypoxemia)
- Increased blood pressure
- Tachycardia (early sign of hypoxemia)

DIFFERENTIAL DIAGNOSIS

Respiratory

- Abnormal airway anatomy
    1. Airway trauma
    2. Malignancy
    3. Mediastinal mass
- Airway obstruction (upper)
- Bronchospasm
- Foreign body (e.g., retained throat pack)
- Neck hematoma
- Pneumothorax/tension pneumothorax

- Subcutaneous emphysema
- Supraglottic or subglottic edema

Other considerations

- Anaphylaxis
- Tension pneumothorax

Diagnostic tests

- Chest X-ray if negative pressure pulmonary edema is suspected

Suggested Readings

- Chen Y, Zhang X. Acute postobstructive pulmonary edema following laryngospasm in elderly patients: a case report. *J Perianesth Nurs*. 2019;34(2):250-258.
- Collins S, Schedler P, Veasey B, Kristofy A, McDowell M. Prevention and treatment of laryngospasm in the pediatric patient: a literature review. *AANA J*. 2019;87(2):145-151.
- Hasoon J, Orhurhu V, Urits I. Negative pressure pulmonary edema following laryngospasm. *Saudi J Anaesth*. 2020;14(2): 265-266.
- Heiner JS. Respiratory anatomy, physiology, pathophysiology, and anesthesia management. In: Elisha S, Heiner JS, Nagelhout JJ, eds. *Nurse Anesthesia*. 7th ed. St. Louis: Elsevier; 2023:615-679.
- Rutt AL, Bojaxhi E, Torp KD. Management of refractory laryngospasm. *J Voice*. 2021;35(4):633-635.

MANAGEMENT

PRIMARY ACTIONS

- Provide supplemental humidified oxygen and increase FiO_2 as needed
- Monitor airway patency, quality of breathing, and hemodynamic stability
- Consult the current American Society of Anesthesiologists Difficult Airway Algorithm for awake intubation and strategies to maintain airway patency
  1. Maintain spontaneous respiration in patients with acute epiglottitis and supraglottitis
  2. Use a smaller than normal external diameter endotracheal tube to minimize tracheal edema in patients with laryngotracheobronchitis
- Provide a calm, nonthreatening environment to prevent anxiety or agitation, which may exacerbate airway resistance and work of breathing
- Secure IV access as the patient's age and condition permits
- Medical management of stridor (see "Medications")

SECONDARY ACTIONS

- Noninvasive supportive ventilation in the adult patient (e.g., continuous positive airway pressure [CPAP] or bilevel positive airway pressure [BiPAP])
- If intubation is required, confirm the presence of an otolaryngologist (ENT surgeon)
  - Maintain spontaneous ventilation during airway management and consider awake intubation
- Consider avoiding neuromuscular blocking agents during intubation (can result in total airway obstruction)
- Extubation should be performed in the OR only after confirmed resolution of supraglottitis

ACUTE EPIGLOTTITIS AND SUPRAGLOTTITIS

Medications

- Glycopyrrolate 2-4 mcg/kg IV bolus (antisialagogue)
- 4% lidocaine solution and 5% lidocaine paste for topical anesthesia for awake intubation (maximum dose 300 mg)
- Ketamine 0.1 to 0.5 mg/kg for sedation and awake intubation in adult
- Ketamine 1 to 2 mg/kg IV bolus (for induction of anesthesia if necessary)
- Antibiotics as appropriate

LARYNGOTRACHEOBRONCHITIS

Medications

- Racemic epinephrine (2.25% solution) 0.05 to 0.1 mL/kg (maximum dose 0.5 mL) nebulization, diluted in 2-3 mL normal saline
- Dexamethasone 0.25-0.5 mg/kg/dose IV for 1 to 3 doses, maximum daily dose 1.5 mg/kg/day
- Heliox (mixture of 70%-80% helium and 20%-30% oxygen)

PHYSIOLOGY/PATHOPHYSIOLOGY

Stridor is a high-pitched inspiratory and expiratory sound caused by turbulent airflow through a partially obstructed upper airway. Stridor may be mechanical (e.g., subglottic edema caused by an endotracheal tube) or pathological, and treatment aims to alleviate the underlying cause. The two distinct pathological processes are associated with similar signs and symptoms, making diagnosis difficult. Acute epiglottitis is inflammation of the epiglottis, and supraglottitis is inflammation and edema of anatomical structures *above* the vocal cords (e.g., edema of the arytenoids and aryepiglottic folds). In contrast, laryngotracheobronchitis involves inflammation and edema of anatomical structures *below* (subglottic) the vocal cords (e.g., trachea, bronchi). Stridor occurs in both the adult and pediatric populations. However, pediatric patients are the most likely to develop complete airway obstruction because of the narrow diameter of their airways. Inflammation significantly increases airway resistance leading to an increased work of breathing and the potential for rapid respiratory failure.

SIGNS AND SYMPTOMS

Neurologic

• Altered level of consciousness
• Anxiety and/or agitation

Respiratory

• Cyanosis
• Desaturation
• High-pitched sound during inspiration and/or expiration
• Hypercarbia
• Hypoxia
• Respiratory arrest
• Substernal retractions
• Tachypnea
• Use of accessory muscles

Cardiovascular

• Bradycardia (late sign)
• Cardiac arrest
• Hypertension (early sign)
• Hypotension (late sign)
• Tachycardia (early sign)

Other considerations

- See Table 6-1 for a comparison of the signs and symptoms that are consistent with epiglottitis/supraglottitis and laryngotracheobronchitis

DIFFERENTIAL DIAGNOSIS

Respiratory

- Airway edema after upper or lower airway surgery
- Airway fire
- Bacterial tracheitis
- Craniofacial and airway abnormalities
- Enlarged tonsils or adenoids
- Foreign body aspiration
- Functional laryngeal dyskinesia
- Laryngeal neoplasm (e.g., laryngeal papillomatosis)
- Laryngeal trauma (e.g., mechanical, chemical, thermal injury)
- Laryngospasm
- Macroglossia
- Peritonsillar abscess

Table 6-1 Comparison of epiglottitis/supraglottitis and laryngotracheobronchitis for the pediatric patient

	ACUTE EPIGLOTTITIS/ SUPRAGLOTTITIS	LARYNGOTRACHEO- BRONCHITIS
Airway obstruction	Supraglottic	Subglottic
Onset of symptoms	Rapid (over 24 h)	Gradual (over 24-72 h)
Pathological cause	Bacterial infection (Haemophilus influenza, Type B)	Viral infection
Most common age group	2-6 years of age	6 mo-6 years of age
Lateral cervical or chest radiograph findings	Enlarged epiglottis (thumbprint sign)	Narrowing of the subglottic area (pencil point or steeple sign)
Laboratory findings	Neutrophilia	Lymphocytosis
Stridor and respiratory phase	Inspiratory phase	Inspiratory and expiratory phase

Continued

Table 6-1 Comparison of epiglottitis/supraglottitis and laryngotracheobronchitis for the pediatric patient—cont'd

	ACUTE EPIGLOTTITIS/ SUPRAGLOTTITIS	LARYNGOTRACHEO- BRONCHITIS
Fever	*High grade (often > 39° C)*	*Low grade (rarely > 39° C)*

Symptoms	• Respiratory distress
	  1. Early signs: agitation, restlessness, tachypnea, tachycardia, and suprasternal or subcostal retractions
	  2. Late signs: lethargy, pallor, cyanosis, sudden cessation of stridor (e.g., total airway obstruction), and hemodynamic collapse
	• Dysphagia and drooling
	• Tripod position: sitting up and leaning forward, which is typical of respiratory distress
		• "Barking" or "brassy" cough
		• Rhinorrhea
		• Respiratory distress presenting with early or late signs

- Pharyngitis
- Postextubation stridor
- Prolonged tracheal intubation
- Retropharyngeal abscess
- Severe tonsillitis
- Spasmodic croup
- Squamous cell carcinoma of the larynx, trachea, or esophagus
- Subglottic hemangioma
- Subglottic stenosis (prolonged intubation, congenital malformation)
- Supraglottic/subglottic edema
- Tracheomalacia/laryngomalacia
- Vocal cord paralysis (e.g., recurrent laryngeal nerve injury)

Cardiovascular

- Vasculitis

Endocrine

- Riedel thyroiditis
- Thyroid goiter

Hematologic

- Angioedema

Musculoskeletal

- Jeune syndrome
- Juvenile rheumatoid arthritis

Other considerations

- Anaphylaxis
- Infectious disease (e.g., diptheria)
- Ludwig angina

Diagnostic tests

- Lateral cervical or chest radiograph

Suggested Readings

- Apfelbaum JL, Hagberg CA, Connis RT, et al. 2022 American Society of Anesthesiologists Practice Guidelines for management of the difficult airway. *Anesthesiology*. 2022;136(1):31-81. doi:10.1097/ALN.0000000000004002.
- Belanger J, Kossick M. Methods of identifying and managing the difficult airway in the pediatric population. *AANA J*. 2015; 83(1):35-41.
- Heiner JS. Airway management. In: Elisha S, Heiner JS, Nagelhout JJ, eds. *Nurse Anesthesia*. 7th ed. St. Louis: Elsevier; 2023:429-476.
- Joyce JA. The other side of the difficult airway: a disciplined, evidence-based approach to emergence and extubation. *AANA J*. 2017;85(1):61-71.

CHAPTER 7   Upper Airway Obstruction

MANAGEMENT

PRIMARY ACTIONS

- Increase FiO_2 to 100%
- Suction airway/endotracheal tube
- Identify and remove obstruction
- Avoid neuromuscular blockade and maintain spontaneous ventilation if possible
- Auscultate bilateral lung fields
  - Manage bronchospasm (See chapter 8 for treatment)
- Reposition the head and neck using head-tilt/chin-lift
- Provide jaw-thrust maneuver
- Insert nasopharyngeal or oropharyngeal airway device
- Consider a supraglottic airway device (e.g., laryngeal mask airway)
- Elevate head of bed to relieve airway compression

SECONDARY ACTIONS

1. Upper airway obstruction caused by a mass or foreign body
   - Maintain spontaneous ventilation
   - Perform an awake intubation with a flexible intubating (fiberoptic) endoscope
     - May consider an awake intubation using video laryngoscope
   - Prepare for emergency cricothyrotomy and have equipment readily available in the event initial airway plans fail
2. Anterior upper mediastinal mass
   - Inquire about radiation or chemotherapy treatments for a mediastinal mass that causes airway obstruction
   - Consider awake intubation using flexible intubating (fiber optic) endoscope if mediastinal mass is in lower trachea
     - Consider using a reinforced endotracheal tube (ETT) or a microlaryngoscopy ETT to bypass distal tracheal compression
     - Use a double lumen ETT for planned single-lung ventilation
   - Change patient position (e.g., semirecumbent, sitting, or lateral) for mediastinal mass that compresses the airway
   - Consider rigid bronchoscopy with jet ventilation for oxygenation and ventilation in acute situations with an inability to advance a flexible intubating (fiber optic) endoscope and/or ETT
   - Place an arterial line in the upper extremity where blood flow is not affected by the mass or
   - If superior vena cava syndrome exists, place an arterial line in the lower extremity
   - Consider cardiopulmonary bypass with a mediastinal mass that can potentially impinge on airway structures

- If superior vena cava syndrome exists, place venous access/ arterial line inferior to the mediastinal mass (e.g., lower extremity)

MEDICATIONS
- Lidocaine 4% for topical anesthesia of the upper airway
- Lidocaine 5% paste for topical anesthesia of the upper airway
- Glycopyrrolate 0.2 mg IV to dry out upper airway secretions
- Epinephrine diluted to 10 mcg/mL
- Sedation for awake intubation (propofol, dexmedetomidine, ketamine, midazolam, or remifentanil)

PHYSIOLOGY AND PATHOPHYSIOLOGY

An airway obstruction can severely decrease or completely block airflow from the upper airway into the lower airway. It can result from a pathologic or pathophysiologic cause, trauma, or even an iatrogenic event, and can occur throughout any time during the perioperative period. This is a broad concept with a variety of factors that can cause this type of crisis.

Obstruction of the upper and/or lower airway leads to impaired ventilation, decreased tissue oxygenation, and diminished removal of carbon dioxide. If hypoxia/hypercarbia ensues, a sympathetic nervous system response will occur in an attempt to increase oxygen delivery to vital organs. Ultimately, if the cause of the airway obstruction is not identified and appropriately managed, then hypoxia will eventually cause cerebral and myocardial demise.

An anterior mediastinal mass can compress the airway and vasculature in the neck or chest depending on where the mass is located. Airway concerns include obstruction of the trachea or lungs, whereas vascular concerns include compression of a subclavian vessel and/or the superior vena cava. If tracheal compression occurs, induction of anesthesia should be performed with extreme caution. The loss of an awake patient's compensatory mechanisms, inability to reposition, paralysis of tracheal and respiratory muscles, and the change from negative to positive pressure ventilation, could lead to complete airway obstruction and even cardiovascular collapse.

SIGNS AND SYMPTOMS

Neurologic
- Altered level of consciousness (e.g., agitation)
- Anxiety

Respiratory

- Accessory muscle use during respiration
- Coughing
- Cyanosis
- Dysphagia
- Dyspnea
- Hemoptysis
- Hypercarbia
- Hypoxemia
- Subcutaneous emphysema
- Tachypnea

UPPER AIRWAY OBSTRUCTION

- Angioedema
- Barky cough
- Burned nose hairs (in cases of fire)
- High peak airway pressure
- Infection
- Skin rash/pruritis (allergic reaction/anaphylaxis)
- Snoring
- Stridor
- Substernal retractions with abdominal "see-saw" type movements
- Tissue trauma
- Tracheal deviation
- Upper airway mass

LOWER AIRWAY OBSTRUCTION

- Abnormal breath sounds during auscultation (e.g., wheezing, rales, or crackles)
- Absence of breath sounds (unilateral or bilateral)
- Flow volume loop abnormalities
- High peak airway pressures
- Infection
- Thoracic or substernal mass
- Tissue trauma

Cardiovascular

- Cardiac dysrhythmias
- Chest pain
- Edema of the face, neck, and upper arms
- Elevated central venous pressure (vena cava syndrome)
- Hypertension/tachycaradia (early signs)
- Hypotension/bradycardia (late signs)

DIFFERENTIAL DIAGNOSIS

Neurologic

- Increased intracranial pressure
- Nerve damage or blockade
    1. Phrenic nerve damage
    2. Recurrent laryngeal nerve damage

Respiratory

- Acute respiratory distress syndrome
- Aspiration
- Atelectasis
- Bronchospasm
- Endotracheal tube malposition/problem
    1. Accidental extubation
    2. Kinking
    3. Mucus plug
    4. Unidentified esophageal intubation
- Laryngeal edema (e.g., postextubation croup)
- Laryngospasm
- Obstructive sleep apnea
- Oral/nasal airway malposition
- Pneumonia
- Pulmonary edema (e.g., congestive heart failure)
- Pulmonary embolism
- Pneumothorax or tension pneumothorax
- Retained pharyngeal/nasopharyngeal packing
- Secretions
- Surgical hematoma
- Tracheomalacia
- Vocal cord polyp

Cardiovascular

- Hypotension

Musculoskeletal

- Congenital craniofacial and airway abnormalities
- Facial, neck, or intrathoracic mass (e.g., thyroid goiter or mediastinal mass)

Pharmacologic

- Anaphylaxis
- Pharmacological considerations:
    1. Alcohol intoxication
    2. Excessive opioid/benzodiazepine/propofol administration
    3. Drug intoxication (e.g., heroin, opioids)

Other considerations

- Circuit disconnect
- Equipment malfunction
    1. Capnography
    2. Pulse oximetry
- Infection
    1. Epiglottitis
    2. Laryngotracheobronchitis
    3. Pneumonia
    4. Tuberculosis
- Trauma (e.g., airway, facial, or thoracic disruption)

Diagnostic tests

- Biopsy of mass
- Pulmonary flow volume loop evaluation
- Radiographic, ultrasound, computed tomography, or magnetic resonance imaging

Suggested Readings

- Erdös G, Tzanova I. Perioperative anaesthetic management of mediastinal mass in adults. *Eur J Anaesthesiol.* 2009;26(8): 627-632.
- Heiner JS. Respiratory anatomy, physiology, pathophysiology, and anesthesia management. In: Elisha S, Heiner JS, Nagelhout JJ, eds. *Nurse Anesthesia.* 7th ed. St. Louis: Elsevier; 2023: 614-679.
- Hillman DR, Platt PR, Eastwood PR. The upper airway during anaesthesia. *Br J Anaesth.* 2003;91(1):31-39.
- Li WW, van Boven WJ, Annema JT, Eberl S, Klomp HM, de Mol BA. Management of large mediastinal masses: surgical and anesthesiological considerations. *J Thorac Dis.* 2016;8(3): E175-E184.
- Lynch J, Crawley SM. Management of airway obstruction. *BJA Educ.* 2018;18(2):46-51.

CHAPTER 8 Bronchospasm

MANAGEMENT

PRIMARY ACTIONS

- Maintain a secure and patent airway
- Administer 100% FiO_2
- Manual ventilation
- Diagnose and treat the underlying cause

MILD TO MODERATE BRONCHOSPASM (patient maintains adequate ventilation with oxygen saturation ≥ 90%)

- Increase anesthetic depth
- Increase inhalational anesthetic concentration
- Administer albuterol (see "Medications")

SEVERE BRONCHOSPASM (difficulty or inability to ventilate, oxygen saturation < 90% with persistent signs and symptoms)

- Call for help
- Stop surgery
- Treatment as indicated above
- Administer epinephrine (see "Medications")

SECONDARY ACTIONS

- Mechanical ventilation—Tidal volume 4-6 mL/kg, adjust the I:E ratio to allow for longer expiratory time
- Arterial blood gas to assess ventilation, acid-base status, and the result of treatment
- Preoperative optimization with bronchodilators for patients with bronchospastic respiratory disease

MEDICATIONS

- Epinephrine 10-100 mcg IV bolus, repeat prn or 0.01 to 0.5 mcg/kg/min IV infusion
- Albuterol 2.5 to 5 mg by nebulization every 20 minutes for three doses, or give 4 to 8 puffs by metered dose inhaler every 20 minutes for 3 doses
- Ipratropium bromide (Atrovent) 500 mcg via nebulizer every 20 minutes for 3 doses, or 4 to 8 puffs by metered dose inhaler every 20 minutes for 3 doses
- Terbutaline 0.25 mg SC injection every 20 minutes times for 3 doses
- Magnesium sulfate 40 to 50 mg/kg IV, or IV infusion of 2 g over 20 minutes
- Hydrocortisone 150 to 200 mg IV
- Aminophylline 6 mg/kg IV loading dose, then 0.5 to 0.7 mg/kg/h infusion

PHYSIOLOGY AND PATHOPHYSIOLOGY

Bronchospasm is an acute and reversible narrowing of the bronchopulmonary segments. Wheezing, a common finding during bronchospasm, results from turbulent airflow through these narrowed segments, causing increased airway resistance. Increased airway reactivity in specific populations (e.g., smoking, chronic obstructive pulmonary disease) may predispose these patients to bronchospastic episodes. During anesthesia, bronchospasm is most often caused by physiologic stimulation (e.g., airway manipulation, endotracheal tube stimulation, surgical stimulation, light anesthesia). Primary treatment includes: (1) maintaining adequate ventilation and oxygenation, (2) increasing anesthetic depth, (3) administering bronchodilators, and (4) identifying and treating the underlying mechanical or pathological cause.

Decreased or sloped (slanted) expiratory limb of the end-tidal carbon dioxide waveform (e.g., "Shark fin" morphology) is characteristic of a mild to moderate bronchospasm due to air trapping from bronchoconstriction, and is shown in Figure 8-1. During severe episodes of bronchospasm, inadequate or the complete inability to ventilate could result in an altered or absent $EtCO_2$ waveform. If this occurs, epinephrine IV is indicated for treatment. As with any disease process, other potential causes (e.g., circuit disconnection or obstructed airway) should be excluded before initiating treatment.

SIGNS AND SYMPTOMS

Respiratory

- Decreased bag compliance during manual ventilation
- Decreased breath sounds
- Desaturation
- Hypercarbia
- Hypoxemia
- Increased peak inspiratory pressure
- Minimal or absent $EtCO_2$/breath sounds (severe bronchospasm)

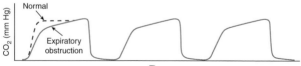

FIGURE 8-1 Sloped expiratory limb on the $EtCO_2$ capnography waveform consistent with bronchospasm

- Sloped expiratory limb on $EtCO_2$ waveform (mild to moderate bronchospasm)
- Wheezing

Cardiovascular

- Cardiac arrest
- Dysrhythmias
- Hypertension
- Tachycardia

DIFFERENTIAL DIAGNOSIS

Respiratory

- Acute gastric aspiration
- Asthma, acute exacerbation
- Chronic obstructive pulmonary disease
- Endotracheal tube contacting the carina or placed in the right mainstem bronchus
- Laryngospasm
- Mechanical airway obstruction
    1. Breathing circuit is obstructed or kinked
    2. Endotracheal tube obstruction (kinking, biting, or mucus plug)
    3. Excessive and thick secretions
- Pneumothorax
- Pulmonary edema
- Pulmonary embolism
- Upper respiratory tract infection with swelling

Pharmacologic

- Airway irritation (e.g., desflurane)
- Anticholinesterase agents
- Beta blockers
- Medications that cause the release of histamine (e.g., atracurium, morphine)
- Nonsteroidal anti-inflammatory drugs (e.g., ketorolac)

Other considerations

- Anaphylaxis
- Carcinoid syndrome
- Endobronchial intubation
- Light anesthesia/surgical stimulation

Diagnostic tests

- Preoperative pulmonary function testing

Suggested Readings

- Baronos S, Selvaraj BJ, Liang M, Ahmed K, Yarmush J. Sugammadex-induced bronchospasm during desflurane anaesthesia. *Br J Anaesth.* 2019;123(1):e155-e156.
- Garcia D, Kehar M, Khan ES, Mendonca R, Girshin M. Multiple episodes of severe bronchospasm during general anesthesia: a case report. *Cureus.* 2022;14(1):e21521.
- Heiner JS. Respiratory anatomy, physiology, pathophysiology, and anesthesia management. In: Elisha S, Heiner JS, Nagelhout JJ, eds. *Nurse Anesthesia.* 7th ed. St. Louis: Elsevier; 2023:615-679.
- Karalapillai D, Weinberg L, Peyton P, et al. Effect of intraoperative low tidal volume vs conventional tidal volume on postoperative pulmonary complications in patients undergoing major surgery: a randomized clinical trial. *JAMA.* 2020;324(9): 848-858.

CHAPTER 9   Hypercarbia

MANAGEMENT

PRIMARY ACTIONS

- Maintain airway, breathing, and circulation
- Provide FiO_2 100%
- Assess the presence and quality of breath sounds
- Assess signs and symptoms associated with hypercarbia
- Identify and treat the definitive cause(s)

SPONTANEOUSLY BREATHING ANESTHETIZED PATIENT:

- Assist with bag-valve-mask ventilation
- Relieve upper airway obstruction (e.g., chin lift, jaw thrust, oral airway)
- Decrease anesthetic depth
- Consider reversal of opioids (naloxone)
- Consider reversal of benzodiazepines (flumazenil)
- Reverse neuromuscular blockade (sugammadex)

MECHANICALLY VENTILATED PATIENT RECEIVING GENERAL ANESTHESIA:

- Confirm correct placement of the airway management device (e.g., laryngeal mask airway, endotracheal tube)
- Increase minute ventilation

SECONDARY INTERVENTIONS

- Obtain arterial blood gas
- Confirm equipment is functioning correctly and consider replacing faulty equipment and/or capnography tubing

PHYSIOLOGY AND PATHOPHYSIOLOGY

Carbon dioxide (CO_2) is a byproduct of cellular metabolism. Hypercarbia is defined as a $PaCO_2 > 45$ mm Hg and occurs because of increased production and/or decreased elimination of CO_2. Central chemoreceptors in the ventrolateral medulla, and peripheral chemoreceptors in the aortic and carotid bodies are sensitive to plasma hydrogen ion and CO_2 conentrations. Excessive CO_2 in the blood will react with water to produce an abundance of hydrogen ions. If the amount of plasma CO_2 reaches extreme levels, the respiratory and renal systems are unable to adequately compensate to decrease hydrogen ion concentrations, and acidosis will occur. The physiologic response to hypercarbia includes sympathetic nervous system hyperactivity resulting in tachycardia, tachypnea, and hypertension.

SIGNS AND SYMPTOMS

Neurologic

• Altered level of consciousness/unconsciousness

Respiratory

• Hypertension
• Increased $EtCO_2$
• Increased $PaCO_2$
• Respiratory acidosis
• Spontaneous respirations during mechanical ventilation
• Tachypnea

Cardiovascular

• Cardiac arrest
• Dysrhythmias
• Tachycardia

Other considerations

• Hyperkalemia

DIFFERENTIAL DIAGNOSIS

Neurologic

• Central nervous system dysfunction
• Hypoglycemia
• Increased intracranial pressure

Respiratory

• Acute gastric aspiration
• Acute respiratory distress syndrome
• Airway obstruction/apnea
• Atelectasis
• Bronchospasm
• Chronic obstructive pulmonary disease
• Endobronchial intubation
• Fractured ribs/pulmonary contusion/diaphragmatic rupture
• Hypoventilation
• Metastatic lung disease
• Pneumothorax/tension pneumothorax
• Positioning (e.g., reverse Trendelenburg, lithotomy positions)
• Postoperative pain during respiration
• Pulmonary edema
• Pulmonary embolism

- Respiratory failure
- Restrictive lung disease (e.g., obesity, pulmonary fibrosis)

Cardiovascular

- Cardiac arrest
- Congestive heart failure
- Dysrhythmias
- Hypotension
- Myocardial ischemia/infarction

Endocrine

- Carcinoid syndrome
- Pheochromocytoma
- Thyrotoxicosis

Musculoskeletal

- Malignant hyperthermia
- Neuromuscular disease (e.g., myasthenia gravis)
- Shivering

Pharmacologic

- Neuroleptic malignant syndrome
- Residual anesthetic medications (e.g., respiratory depressants, neuromuscular blocking drugs)
- Salicylate toxicity

Other considerations

- Anesthesia machine malfunction
  1. Exhausted CO_2 absorbent (increased $FiCO_2$)
  2. Inspiratory or expiratory valve malfunction
  3. Kinked or obstructed breathing circuit or endotracheal tube
- Electrolyte abnormality
- Esophageal intubation
- Hyperthermia
- Infection/sepsis
- Massive hemorrhage
- Reperfusion of ischemic tissue (e.g., removal of the aortic cross cross-clamp, deflation of thigh cuff)
- Subcutaneous emphysema
- Systemic absorption of CO_2 during laparoscopic surgery

Diagnostic tests

- Arterial blood gas
- Chest X-ray

Suggested Readings

- Aldakhil SK, Tashkandi AA, Al Harbi MK, Al Shehri A. Subcutaneous emphysema and hypercarbia as a complication of laparoscopic procedure: case report. *J Surg Case Rep*. 2020;2020(3): rjz415. doi:10.1093/jscr/rjz415.
- Atkinson TM, Giraud GD, Togioka BM, Jones DB, Cigarroa JE. Cardiovascular and ventilatory consequences of laparoscopic surgery. *Circulation*. 2017;135(7):700-710.
- Heiner JS. Respiratory anatomy, physiology, pathophysiology, and anesthesia management. In: Elisha S, Heiner JS, Nagelhout JJ, eds. *Nurse Anesthesia*. 7th ed. St. Louis: Elsevier; 2023:615-679.
- Merle E, Zaatari S, Spiegel R. Is it the pH that matters? Challenging the pathophysiology of acidemia in a case of severe hypercapnia secondary to intraoperative CO_2 insufflation. *Case Rep Crit Care*. 2020;2020:1898759. doi:10.1155/2020/1898759.

CHAPTER 10   Hypoxia

MANAGEMENT

PRIMARY ACTIONS

- Administer 100% oxygen
- Determine and treat the specific cause of hypoxia (see Table 10-1)
- Manual ventilation/confirm airway patency—ausculation, bilateral chest rise and fall, continuous $EtCO_2$ waveform
- Rapidly verify pulse oximetry reading with adequate plethysmography
- Endotracheal intubation/confirm correct placement with $EtCO_2$ waveform capnography and/or visual confirmation with videolaryngoscope or flexible intubating bronchoscope
  - Consider supraglottic airway placement if needed
- Obtain arterial blood gas
- Administer bronchodilators as needed
- Consider continuous positive airway pressure if the patient is not intubated
- Consider positive end-expiratory pressure if patient is intubated
- Perform cardiac resuscitation per American Heart Association ACLS/PALS protocol as necessary

SECONDARY ACTIONS

- Communicate assessment and plan with health care team
- Consider suctioning trachea, corticosteroid, and/or antibiotics for gastric aspiration (See Chapter 2 for treatment of gastric aspiration)
- Descend to lower elevation for high-altitude hypoxia
- Consider vasopressors and inotropes for stagnant hypoxia depending on cause (see "Medications")
- 100% FiO_2 and/or hyperbaric oxygen therapy for carbon monoxide or cyanide poisoning
- Contact poison control for cyanide poisoning (www.poison.org)
- Consider hydroxocobalamin or sodium thiosulfate for cyanide poisoning (see "Medications")

MEDICATIONS

- Albuterol by nebulizer 2.5 to 5 mg
- Vasopressor(s) to maintain mean arterial pressure >65 mm Hg for cardiovascular and shock issues:
  - Ephedrine 5 to 10 mg IV bolus and/or,
  - Phenylephrine 50 to 100 mcg IV bolus, 0.1 to 0.5 mcg/kg/min infusion and/or,
  - Epinephrine 10 to 100 mcg IV bolus, 0.1 to 0.5 mcg/kg/min infusion and/or,
  - Dopamine 5 to 20 mcg/kg/min IV infusion and/or,

- Norepinephrine 5 to 10 mcg IV bolus, 0.1 to 0.5 mcg/kg/min infusion and/or,
- Vasopressin 1-2 Unit IV bolus, 0.01 to 0.05 Units/min infusion
- For administration of hydroxocobalamin or sodium thiosulfate consult an in-house pharmacist:
  - Hydroxocobalamin starting dose 5 g IV infusion over 15 minutes (15 mL/min)
  - Sodium thiosulfate 12.5 g IV infusion over 10 minutes

PHYSIOLOGY AND PATHOPHYSIOLOGY

Hypoxemia is defined as a low blood oxygen content and is assessed by an SpO_2 <90% or PaO_2 <60 mm Hg. Hypoxia primarily results from hypoxemia and is defined as a low oxygen supply at the body tissue cellular level. Oxygen is a vital component necessary for cellular metabolism and energy (adenosine triphosphate) production. When oxygen concentrations are decreased, anaerobic metabolism follows resulting in cellular dysfunction, acidosis, multiorgan system failure, and eventually death. Hypoxia is divided into four categories: (1) anemic hypoxia, (2) hypoxic hypoxia, (3) stagnant hypoxia, and (4) histotoxic hypoxia. Possible causes of hypoxia are included in Table 10-1.

Anemic hypoxia refers to any condition that affects the production or function of the red blood cell and hemoglobin molecule. Hypoxic hypoxia indicates conditions that impair or decrease oxygen from reaching the lungs and subsequent diffusion into the blood. Stagnant hypoxia is any disorder that leads to inadequate tissue oxygenation from a reduction in blood flow. Finally, histotoxic hypoxia causes impaired oxygen usage at the cellular level, specifically the inhibition of cytochrome oxidase.

In the neonatal population, the sympathetic nervous system is functionally immature resulting in parasympathetic nervous system predominance; the ensuing physical signs associated

Table 10-1 Types and causes of hypoxia

ANEMIC HYPOXIA
• Carbon monoxide poisoning
• Chemotherapy
• Hemorrhage
• Renal disease
• Sickle cell disease
• Thalassemia

Table 10-1 Types and causes of hypoxia—cont'd

HYPOXIC HYPOXIA
- Alterations in nerve transmission (e.g., neurogenic shock, recurrent laryngeal nerve injury, phrenic nerve dysfunction, local anesthetic induced nerve blockade)
- CNS depression (e.g., medications, trauma, hypoperfusion)
- Decreased FiO_2 (e.g., absence of ventilation, hypoxic mixture, high altitude)
- Decreased functional residual capacity (e.g., obesity, pregnancy, restrictive lung disease)
- Equipment malfunction (e.g., circuit leak or disconnection, kink in endotracheal tube, pipeline failure)
- Obstructive lung disease (e.g., chronic obstructive pulmonary disease, asthma)
- Respiratory muscle incompetency or failure (e.g., diaphragmatic trauma, high spinal anesthetic)
- Thoracic structural malformations (e.g., scoliosis, thoracic trauma)

Upper airway conditions:
- Foreign body
- Laryngospasm
- Mass/thyroid goiter
- Obstructive sleep apnea
- Upper respiratory tract infection

Lower airway conditions:
- Inflammation (e.g., acute respiratory distress syndrome, cystic fibrosis)
- Pneumothorax/hemothorax/tension pneumothorax
- Pneumonia
- Pulmonary contusion
- Restrictive/obstructive lung disease

Increased dead space ventilation:
- Pulmonary embolism
- Pulmonary vasoconstriction

Increased intrapulmonary shunt:
- Aspiration with direct bronchiolar and alveolar tissue damage
- Atelectasis
- Bronchospasm
- Pulmonary edema

STAGNANT HYPOXIA
- Polycythemia
- Pump failure (e.g., congestive heart failure, myocardial infarction, trauma, cardiac tamponade)
- Severe hypotension (e.g., hemorrhage, sepsis, anaphylaxis, neurogenic shock)

Continued

Table 10-1 Types and causes of hypoxia—cont'd

HISTOTOXIC HYPOXIA
• Alcohol poisoning
• Carbon monoxide poisoning
• Cyanide poisoning
• Hydrogen sulfide poisoning

with hypoxia in this population may include respiratory arrest, bradycardia, and cardiac arrest.

SIGNS AND SYMPTOMS

Neurologic

- Agitation
- Altered level of consciousness
- Altered nerve transmission (e.g., recurrent laryngeal nerve injury, phrenic nerve paralysis with reduced diaphragmatic contraction)
- Headache
- Nausea and/or vomiting
- Seizures
- Somnolence leading to unconsciousness

Respiratory

- Altered or absent $EtCO_2$ waveform
- Cyanosis
- Decreased, abnormal (e.g., wheezing, crackles, rales), or absent breath sounds
- Decreased arterial oxygen (PaO_2 <60 mm Hg)
- Decreased pulse oximetry reading (SpO_2 <90%)
- Elevated methemoglobin/carboxyhemoglobin levels
- High peak airway pressures
- Hypoventilation
- Pallor
- Respiratory rate:
    - Early sign – tachypnea
    - Late sign – bradypnea/apnea
- Stridor
- Tachypnea

Cardiovascular

- Early signs:
    1. Hypertension
    2. Tachycardia

- Late signs:
  1. Bradycardia
  2. Hypotension

Musculoskeletal

- Visual assessment of altered anatomy of the airway or chest

Other considerations

- Active hemorrhage
- Anesthesia machine alarms for low flow or circuit disconnect
- Low FiO_2
- Trauma to the airway

DIFFERENTIAL DIAGNOSIS

Respiratory

- Airway fire
- Airway obstruction
- Aspiration
- Atelectasis
- Bronchospasm
- Decreased FiO_2 administration (e.g., hypoxic mixture, high altitude)
- Decreased functional residual capacity (e.g., obesity, pregnancy)
- Esophageal/endobronchial intubation
- Hypoventilation (e.g., residual anesthetic effects, inadequate ventilation settings)
- Hypoxic pulmonary vasoconstriction inhibition
- Interstitial lung disease
- Intrapulmonary shunt
- Obstructive lung disease (e.g., asthma, chronic obstructive pulmonary disease)
- Pneumonia
- Pneumothorax
- Pulmonary edema
- Pulmonary embolism
- Smoke inhalation
- Traumatic lung injury

Cardiovascular

- Intracardiac shunt
- Myocardial ischemia/infarction

Neurologic

- Cerebral herniation
- Neuromuscular disorder (e.g., myasthenia gravis, Parkinson exacerbation, multiple sclerosis, Guillain Barré syndrome)

Endocrine

- Acute pancreatitis
- Pheochromocytoma

Hematologic

- Transfusion reaction from blood product administration

Hepatic

- Liver disease

Musculoskeletal

- External airway compression (e.g., thyroid tumor)
- Hypermetabolic states (e.g., malignant hyperthermia, thyrotoxicosis)
- Structural abnormalities (e.g., scoliosis, thoracic cage malformations)

Pharmacologic

- Alcohol intoxication
- Central nervous system depressants (e.g., opioids, benzodiazepines, barbiturates, marijuana)
- Cyanide poisoning (e.g., sodium nitroprusside infusions, smoke inhalation, chemicals in the workplace)
- Local anesthetic toxicity
- Methylene blue or indigo carmine

Other considerations

- All shock states
- Anesthesia machine failure
- Carbon monoxide poisoning
- Equipment malfunction (e.g., pulse oximetry, mass spectrometry, anesthesia machine malfunction)
- Type of surgical procedure (e.g., pneumonectomy, thoracic surgery, cardiac surgery)

diagnostic tests

- Electrocardiogram
- Arterial blood gas
- Chest X-ray
- Transesophageal echocardiogram
- Hemoglobin and hematocrit

Suggested Readings

- Bhutta BS, Alghoula F, Berim I. Hypoxia. [Updated 2022 Feb 9]. In: *StatPearls* [Internet]. Treasure Island, FL: StatPearls Publishing; 2022. Available at: https://www.ncbi.nlm.nih.gov/books/NBK482316/.
- Heiner JS. Respiratory anatomy, physiology, pathophysiology, and anesthesia management. In: Elisha S, Heiner JS, Nagelhout JJ, eds. *Nurse Anesthesia*. 7th ed. St. Louis: Elsevier; 2023:614-679.
- Kane AD, Kothmann E, Giussani DA. Detection and response to acute systemic hypoxia. *BJA Educ*. 2020;20(2):58-64. doi:10.1016/j.bjae.2019.10.004.
- Leach RM, Treacher DF. Oxygen transport-2. Tissue hypoxia. *BMJ*. 1998;317(7169):1370-1373.
- Odom-Foreren J, Brady JM. Postanesthesia recovery. In: Elisha S, Heiner JS, Nagelhout JJ, eds. *Nurse Anesthesia*. 7th ed. St. Louis: Elsevier; 2023:1282-1283.
- Sarkar M, Niranjan N, Banyal PK. Mechanisms of hypoxemia [published correction appears in Lung India. 2017;34(2):220]. *Lung India*. 2017;34(1):47-60.

CHAPTER 11   Pneumothorax, Hemothorax, and Tension Pneumothorax

MANAGEMENT

PRIMARY ACTIONS

- Administer 100% oxygen
- Call for help
- Maintain airway patency (e.g., endotracheal intubation)
- Convert to manual ventilation if patient is receiving mechanical ventilation
  - Use with caution and avoid excessive inspiratory pressures
  - If the patient is spontaneously breathing, avoid positive pressure ventilation until the chest tube is in place
- Needle decompression (if patient is hemodynamically unstable) on affected side
  - Large-bore IV placed at second intercostal space in the mid-clavicular line above the rib
- Chest tube placement on affected side, with chest X-ray to confirm placement

SECONDARY ACTIONS

- Avoid nitrous oxide
- Cover penetrating chest wound with an airtight occlusive bandage and clean plastic sheeting
- Monitor and treat anemia and hypovolemia in the event of hemothorax (consider volume replacement and blood product administration)
- Obtain arterial blood gas (ABG)
- Obtain chest radiograph and chest computed tomography scan
- Obtain complete blood count and coagulation studies
- Assisted ventilation strategy after chest tube placement:
  1. Low volume to avoid volutrauma (4-6 mL/kg)
  2. Adjust respiratory rate to maintain normocapnia
  3. Minimize peak airway pressures to avoid barotrauma (< 30 cm H_2O)
  4. Use of low positive end-expiratory pressure (5-10 cm H_2O)
- For unresolving pneumothorax consult thoracic surgeon for possible video-assisted thoracoscopic surgery

PHYSIOLOGY AND PATHOPHYSIOLOGY

A pneumothorax occurs when air becomes trapped within the pleural space, eliminating the pressure gradient between the negative plural space and the intrapulmonary space. The removal of this pressure gradient leads to compression of the affected lung, respiratory distress, and hypoxemia. A pneumothorax can result from a disruption and opening between the alveoli and pleural spaces, exposure of the pleural space to atmospheric air, or on rare occasions, the presence of an anaerobic gas-producing organism. There are four possible causes of pneumothorax, including:

(1) Trauma: blunt, penetrating trauma, and rib fracture
(2) Spontaneous: weakened pulmonary parenchyma (e.g., chronic obstructive pulmonary disease with emphysematous bullae or blebs)
(3) Iatrogenic: complication of central line placement, volutrauma, barotrauma, biotrauma, and atelectrauma
(4) Infectious: tuberculosis or pleural effusion

A tension pneumothorax develops when tissue at the site of the injury acts as a one-way valve into the thoracic cavity. During inspiration, air becomes trapped within the pleural space and does not escape during expiration. The accumulation of air within the pleural space increases intrathoracic pressure, which: (1) dramatically compresses the affected (ipsilateral) lung; (2) prevents effective diaphragmatic contraction; and (3) exerts pressure on the mediastinal structures and contralateral lung. This intrathoracic pressure shifts the mediastinum toward the contralateral lung, compressing the heart and lung tissue resulting in reduced cardiac output and added respiratory distress. A tension pneumothorax is a medical emergency that requires prompt identification and management.

A hemothorax occurs as a result of blood accumulating within the pleural space. Trauma, infection, or iatrogenic mechanisms can cause vascular damage and rupture, resulting in hemorrhage into the pleural cavity. A hemopneumothorax is the combination of pneumothorax and hemothorax (e.g., air and blood within the pleural space). This pathophysiologic process may progress to tension hemopneumothorax, resulting in compression of the mediastinum and subsequent cardiac and respiratory decompensation.

SIGNS AND SYMPTOMS

Neurologic

• Altered level of consciousness

Respiratory

• Absent or decreased breath sounds on affected side
• Cyanosis
• Decreased or altered $EtCO_2$ (tension pneumothorax and decreased cardiac output)
• Dyspnea
• Hemoptysis (hemothorax)
• Hypoxemia – SpO_2 <90%, PaO_2 < 60 mm Hg
• Increased $EtCO_2/PaCO_2$
• Increased peak airway pressure
• Pallor
• Paradoxical respiration
• Possible contusion, bruising, abrasion, or laceration on affected side
• Radiographic translucency on affected side
• Subcutaneous emphysema
• Tachypnea
• Tracheal deviation away from affected side in tension pneumothorax

Cardiovascular

• Chest pain
• Hypertension (early sign)
• Hypotension (late sign)
• Jugular venous distention (may be seen in tension pneumothorax)
• Narrowed pulse pressure
• Potential cardiovascular collapse after initiation of positive pressure ventilation (tension pneumothorax)
• Tachycardia

Other considerations

• Central venous line placement with trauma to the lung
• Existence of emphysematous bullae or blebs
• Intrathoracic surgeries
• Inferior displacement of diaphragm (may be noted by surgeon during laparoscopy)
• Subcutaneous emphysema on the chest and neck
• Surgical manipulation of areas close to the parietal pleura
• Trauma to the chest (blunt or penetrating)

DIFFERENTIAL DIAGNOSIS

Respiratory

- Atelectasis
- Bronchospasm
- Chronic obstructive pulmonary disease
- Empyema
- Hypoventilation
- Pneumonia
- Pulmonary embolism

Cardiovascular

- Acute coronary syndrome
- Acute pericarditis
- Cardiac tamponade
- Intraoperative hemodynamic instability
- Myocardial infarction

Musculoskeletal

- Costochondritis
- Diaphragmatic injury
- Intercostal muscle spasm
- Obesity or excessive chest tissue leading to inability to auscultate breath sounds
- Rib fracture

Other considerations

- Anaphylaxis
- Esophageal spasm
- Equipment malfunction (e.g., pulse oximetry, mass spectrometry)

Diagnostic tests

- Baseline ABG and subsequent ABG for comparison
- Baseline chest X-ray and subsequent ABG for comparison
- Chest auscultation
- Chest computed tomography
- Coagulation studies (prothrombin time, partial thromboplastin time, international normalized ratio, thromboelastography)
- Consult thoracic surgeon, pulmonologist, interventional radiologist, and intensivist
- Hemoglobin/hematocrit
- Point of care ultrasound of the chest
  - Pneumothorax confirmed using a high-frequency linear transducer probe observing for four sonographic signs: (1) the presence of lung point, (2) absence of lung sliding, (3) absence

of B-lines, and (4) absence of lung pulse (lack of cardiophasic movement of a fully inflated lung at the visceral parietal pleura)

Suggested Readings

- Heiner JS. Respiratory anatomy, physiology, pathophysiology, and anesthesia management. In: Elisha S, Heiner JS, Nagelhout JJ, eds. *Nurse Anesthesia*. 7th ed. St. Louis: Elsevier; 2023:614-679.
- Fiza B, Moll V, Ferrero N. The lung point: early identification of pneumothorax on point of care ultrasound. *Anesthesiology*. 2019;131:1148.
- Jalota Sahota R, Sayad E. Tension pneumothorax. [Updated 2021 Aug 11]. In: *StatPearls* [Internet]. Treasure Island, FL: StatPearls Publishing; 2022. Available at: https://www.ncbi.nlm.nih.gov/books/NBK559090/.
- Khalil PA, Merelman A, Riccio J, et al. Randomized controlled trial of point-of-care ultrasound education for the recognition of tension pneumothorax by paramedics in prehospital simulation. *Prehosp Disaster Med*. 2021;36(1):74-78.
- Oh SK, Cho SI, Won YJ, Yun JH. Bilateral tension pneumothorax during endoscopic submucosal dissection under general anesthesia diagnosed by point-of-care ultrasound — a case report. *Anesth Pain Med (Seoul)*. 2021;16(2):171-176.
- Roberts DJ, Leigh-Smith S, Faris PD, et al. Clinical presentation of patients with tension pneumothorax: a systematic review. *Ann Surg*. 2015;261(6):1068-1078

CHAPTER 12 Autonomic Hyperreflexia

MANAGEMENT

PRIMARY ACTIONS

- Notify the surgeon and stop the procedure if necessary
- Check for bowel, bladder, or uterine distention
- Eliminate noxious stimulus below the spinal cord injury
- Administer 100% FiO_2
- Increase anesthetic depth
- Position head up (e.g., reverse Trendelenburg)
- Administer one or more antihypertensive medications and titrate to the patient's pre-crisis blood pressure (see "Medications")

SECONDARY ACTIONS

- Invasive monitoring (e.g., arterial line, central venous catheter)
- Manage neurologic, cardiac, and pulmonary manifestations associated with hypertension
- Neuraxial anesthesia (e.g., epidural anesthesia) if uterine contractions cause autonomic hyperreflexia

MEDICATIONS

- Antihypertensives
  - Nicardipine 0.2 to 0.5 mg IV bolus, 2.5 to 15 mg/h infusion and/or,
  - Nitroglycerin 5 to 100 mcg/min IV infusion and/or,
  - Nitroprusside 0.2 to 5 mcg/kg/min IV infusion and/or,
  - Hydralazine 5 mg IV bolus every 10 minutes, up to 20 mg total dose and/or,
  - Labetalol 5 mg IV bolus every 5 minutes, up to 50 mg total dose

PHYSIOLOGY AND PATHOPHYSIOLOGY

Autonomic hyperreflexia, or dysreflexia, describes the sudden sympathetic nervous system response that occurs after chronic spinal cord injury. It occurs in up to 85% of patients with spinal cord injury above the T6 vertebral level. The classic presentation of autonomic hyperreflexia includes systemic hypertension, bradycardia, and cutaneous vasodilation above the level of the spinal cord injury.

Noxious stimulation below the level of the spinal cord injury activates sensory impulses, which stimulate a sympathetic nervous system response, vasoconstriction of the splanchnic circulation, and an increase in systemic blood pressure. Higher neurological centers modulate this sympathetic response in neurologically intact patients. However, complete spinal cord transection isolates neurological modulation from the sympathetic response, and vasoconstriction persists below the level of the injury. Increased systemic vascular resistance with resulting hypertension activates central and peripheral baroreceptors. Bradycardia and cutaneous vasodilation subsequently occur above the level of spinal cord transection.

SIGNS AND SYMPTOMS

Neurologic

- Altered level of consciousness
- Blurred vision
- Cerebral herniation
- Cerebral vascular accident
- Headache
- Intracranial hemorrhage
- Seizures

Respiratory

- Hypoxemia
- Nasal congestion
- Pulmonary edema

Cardiovascular

- Cardiac dysrhythmias
- Classic presentation
  1. Bradycardia
  2. Cutaneous vasodilation above the level of the spinal cord transection (e.g., piloerection, sweating, nasal congestion, cutaneous flushing)
  3. Systemic hypertension
- Congestive heart failure
- Myocardial infarction or ischemia

DIFFERENTIAL DIAGNOSIS

Neurologic

- Increased intracranial pressure (e.g., Cushing reflex)
  1. Intracranial neoplasm
  2. Neurovascular pathology
  3. Traumatic brain injury

- Neuroleptic malignant syndrome
- Noxious stimulus below the level of spinal cord transection
  1. Cutaneous or visceral stimulation (e.g., surgery, temperature extremes)
  2. Distension of a hollow organ (e.g., bowel, bladder, uterus)
  3. Intense smooth muscle contraction (e.g., uterine contractions)

Cardiovascular

- Essential hypertension
- Myocardial infarction

Endocrine

- Carcinoid syndrome
- Pheochromocytoma
- Thyrotoxicosis

Pharmacologic

- Acute drug intoxication (e.g., stimulants, cocaine, amphetamines)
- Anticholinergic toxicity
- Cholinergic crisis
- Medication error such as excessive adrenergic receptor agonist administration (e.g., phenylephrine, epinephrine)
- Serotonin syndrome

Other considerations

- Inadequate depth of anesthesia
- Malignant hyperthermia
- Preeclampsia or eclampsia in a parturient with spinal cord transection

Suggested Readings

- Conley A, Biddle C, Baker K. A tour of autonomic reflex activity relevant to clinical practice. *AANA J.* 2017;85(2):141-147.
- Eldahan KC, Rabchevsky AG. Autonomic dysreflexia after spinal cord injury: systemic pathophysiology and methods of management. *Auton Neurosci.* 2018;209:59-70. doi:10.1016/j.autneu.2017.05.002.
- Rao S, Treggiari MM. Anesthesia for acute spinal cord injury. *Anesthesiol Clin.* 2021;39(1):127-138. doi:10.1016/j.anclin.2020.11.011.

CHAPTER 13   Cardiac Dysrhythmias

MANAGEMENT

PRIMARY ACTIONS

- Identify the presence of cardiac dysrhythmia in two leads (e.g., II and V5)
- Treat hypoxemia or hypercarbia
- Assess for hemodynamic instability: altered level of consciousness, hypotension, respiratory arrest, or loss of peripheral/central pulses
- Follow current ACLS/PALS guidelines
- See Table 13-1 for management of specific cardiac dysrhythmias (see "Medications")
- Treat underlying pathological causes

SECONDARY ACTIONS

- Supportive measures as necessary (see "Medications")
  1. Airway management and mechanical ventilation
  2. Invasive monitoring (e.g., arterial, central venous catheter)
  3. Monitor acid-base, fluid, and electrolyte balance
- Consult with cardiologist

MEDICATIONS (follow current ACLS/PALS guidelines for timing and dosing of medications)

- Antidysrhythmics:
  - Amiodarone intial dose: 300 mg IV bolus; for refractory VT/VF may repeat with 150 mg IV bolus at 5 to 10 min intervals; after conversion begin 360 mg IV infusion for 6 hours (1 mg/min); maximum dose is 2.2. gm in 24 hours; or
  - Lidocaine Initial dose: 1 to 1.5 mg/kg IV bolus; for refractory VT/VF may repeat with 0.5 to 0.75 mg/kg IV bolus at 5 to 10 minute intervals; maximum 3 doses or total of 3 mg/kg.
  - Diltiazem 0.25 to 0.35 mg/kg IV bolus or,
  - Esmolol 500 mcg/kg IV bolus, 50 mcg/kg/min infusion
- Vasopressor(s) to maintain mean arterial pressure >65 mm Hg:
  - Ephedrine 5 to 10 mg IV bolus and/or,
  - Phenylephrine 50 to 100 mcg IV bolus, 0.1 to 0.5 mcg/kg/min infusion and/or,
  - **Epinephrine 10 to 100 mcg IV bolus, 0.1 to 0.5 mcg/kg/min infusion and/or,**
  - Dopamine 5 to 20 mcg/kg/min IV infusion and/or,
  - Norepinephrine 5 to 10 mcg IV bolus, 0.1 to 0.5 mcg/kg/min infusion and/or,
  - Vasopressin 1 to 4 Units IV bolus, 0.01 to 0.1 Units/min infusion

PHYSIOLOGY AND PATHOPHYSIOLOGY

During a normal cardiac cycle, the heart's conduction pathways and structural components work in coordination. Cardiac synchrony is vital for oxygen delivery to peripheral and central tissues. Cardiac dysrhythmias disrupt this synchrony and can compromise cardiac output to vital organs. Causes of cardiac dysrhythmias include physiologic stress, myocardial oxygen demand exceeding supply, and cardiac conduction or structural abnormalities.

Medical management may include antidysrhythmic medication, antithrombotic medication, direct current cardioversion, and/or intracardiac device placement (e.g., pacemaker, automatic implantable cardioverter-defibrillator). The specific treatment of cardiac dysrhythmias should be based on managing the underlying pathological state and instituting ACLS or PALS guidelines. See Table 13-1 for symptoms, differential diagnosis, and treatment for the following cardiac dysrhythmias:
• Sinus bradycardia and atrioventricular (AV) heart block
• Sinus tachycardia

Table 13-1 Cardiac dysrhythmias: symptoms, differential diagnosis, and treatment

CARDIAC DYSRHYTHMIAS	SIGNS AND SYMPTOMS	DIFFERENTIAL DIAGNOSIS	TREATMENT
Bradycardia	• Sinus bradycardia HR < 60 BPM • First-, second-, third-degree AV nodal block	• Conduction disease • Structural disease • Perioperative stress • ACLS Hs and 5 Ts*	• ACLS or PALS • Atropine • Transcutaneous pacing • Dopamine • Epinephrine
Tachycardia	• Sinus tachycardia HR > 100 BPM	• Conduction disease • Structural disease • Perioperative stress • ACLS Hs and 5 Ts*	• Increase depth of anesthesia • Provide analgesia • Assess for hypovolemia • Assess for a hypermetabolic pathological state

Continued

Table 13-1 Cardiac dysrhythmias: symptoms, differential diagnosis, and treatment—cont'd

CARDIAC DYSRHYTHMIAS	SIGNS AND SYMPTOMS	DIFFERENTIAL DIAGNOSIS	TREATMENT
Atrial Tachydysrhythmias	• Atrial fibrillation and flutter • Supraventricular tachycardia	• Conduction disease • Structural disease • Perioperative stress • 8 Hs and 8 Ts*	• ACLS or PALS **Atrial fibrillation and flutter treatment** • Echocardiography to rule out atrial thrombus • Synchronized cardioversion • Rate control with diltiazem, beta blockers, or digoxin **SVT treatment** • Vagal maneuvers (eg, Valsalva maneuver) • Rate control with adenosine, diltiazem, beta blockers (see "Medications")

Table 13-1 Cardiac dysrhythmias: symptoms, differential diagnosis, and treatment—cont'd

CARDIAC DYSRHYTHMIAS	SIGNS AND SYMPTOMS	DIFFERENTIAL DIAGNOSIS	TREATMENT
Ventricular tachydysrhythmias	• Ventricular tachycardia and fibrillation • Torsades de pointes	• Conduction disease • Structural disease • Perioperative stress • 8 Hs and 8 Ts*	• ACLS or PALS • ACLS or PALS **Ventricular tachycardia and fibrillation treatment** • Biphasic defibrillation • Epinephrine • Vasopressin • Amiodarone • Lidocaine **Torsades de Pointes treatment** • Treatment as above • Consider magnesium sulfate
PEA and asystole	• PEA • Asystole	• Conduction disease • Structural disease • Perioperative stress • 8 Hs and 8 Ts*	• ACLS or PALS • Epinephrine • Vasopressin • Atropine

Abbreviations: BPM, beats/min; HR, heart rate; PEA, pulseless electrical activity.
*See the Differential Diagnosis section for Hs and Ts.

- Atrial tachyarrhythmias (e.g., atrial fibrillation, atrial flutter, supraventricular tachycardia)
- Ventricular tachyarrhythmias (e.g., ventricular tachycardia, ventricular fibrillation, Torsades de pointes)
- Pulseless electrical activity and asystole

SIGNS AND SYMPTOMS

Neurologic

- Altered level of consciousness/loss of consciousness
- Ischemic stroke

Respiratory

- Hypoxemia
- Hypercarbia
- Pulmonary edema

Cardiovascular

- Cardiac dysrhythmia in two leads (e.g., II and V5)
- Chest pain
- Congestive heart failure
- Hypotension
- Left ventricular dysfunction
- Loss of peripheral/central pulses
- Myocardial ischemia or infarction

Gastrointestinal

- Nausea and/or vomiting

DIFFERENTIAL DIAGNOSIS

Cardiovascular

- Conduction cardiac disease
  1. First-, second-, or third-degree AV nodal block
  2. Fascicular block (bundle branch block)
  3. Q-T interval prolongation
  4. Sinus node dysfunction (e.g., sick sinus syndrome)
  5. Wolff-Parkinson-White syndrome
- Structural cardiac disease
  1. Cardiomyopathy (e.g., concentric or eccentric)
  2. Cardiopulmonary disease (e.g., chronic obstructive pulmonary disease)
  3. Congenital cardiac disease
  4. Coronary artery disease
  5. Inflammatory disease (e.g., pericarditis)
  6. Postcardiac surgical intervention
  7. Valvular cardiac disease

Other considerations

- Perioperative physiologic stress
  1. Induction and emergence of anesthesia
  2. Neuraxial anesthesia (e.g., sympathectomy, high spinal anesthesia)
  3. Laryngoscopy and tracheal intubation
  4. Inadequate depth of anesthesia and analgesia
  5. Surgical stimulation and pain
  6. Medication overdose or error

- ACLS Hs
  1. Hydrogen ion excess (e.g., hypercarbia, acidosis)
  2. Hyper-/hypo-electrolyte abnormalities (e.g., sodium, potassium, calcium, magnesium)
  3. Hypervagal (e.g., parasympathetic predominance)
  4. Hyperthermia (e.g., malignant hyperthermia)
  5. Hypoglycemia
  6. Hypothermia
  7. Hypovolemia
  8. Hypoxia
- ACLS Ts
  1. Tablets (e.g., digitalis, droperidol, other medication overdoses)
  2. Tamponade, cardiac
  3. Tension (e.g., tension pneumothorax, pulmonary hypertension)
  4. Thrombosis (e.g., pulmonary embolus, coronary with myocardial infarction)
  5. Thyroid (e.g., myxedema coma, thyrotoxicosis)
  6. Toxicity (e.g., anaphylaxis, local anesthetic toxicity)
  7. Trauma (e.g., shock states)
  8. Treatment, cancer (e.g., doxorubicin)
- See Table 13-1 for signs and symptoms, differential diagnosis, and treatment of specific cardiac dysrhythmias

Diagnostic tests

- 12-lead electrocardiogram
- Arterial blood gas
- Echocardiogram (e.g., transthoracic, transesophageal)
- Serum electrolyte test(s): sodium, potassium, calcium, and magnesium
- Transthoracic ultrasound

Suggested Readings

- Elisha S, Heiner J, Nagelhout J, Gabot M. Venous thromboembolism: new concepts in perioperative management. *AANA J.* 2015;83(3):211-221.
- Khan ZH, Movafegh A, Ali HKA. Dysrhythmias under general anesthesia and their management. *Arch Anesthesiol Crit Care.* 2019;5(3):104-106.
- Kwon CH, Kim SH. Intraoperative management of critical arrhythmia. *Korean J Anesthesiol.* 2017;70(2):120-126.

MANAGEMENT

PRIMARY ACTIONS (FOR ALL TYPES OF EMBOLI)
- Call for help
- Administer 100% oxygen
- Discontinue anesthetic agents
- IV fluid bolus
- Administer vasopressor(s) for hypotension (see "Medications")
- Endotracheal intubation if respiratory distress occurs
- Invasive monitoring (arterial and or central venous catheter) as necessary
- Consider transesophageal echocardiography
- Perform ACLS/PALS per American Heart Association protocol

VENOUS AIR EMBOLISM: NOTIFY SURGEON/FLOOD THE SURGICAL FIELD

CO$_2$ GAS EMBOLISM: NOTIFY THE SURGEON/REMOVE THE PNEUMOPERITONEUM
- Reposition in left lateral decubitus position and move operative site below the level of the heart
- Aspirate the embolism from the distal port of a central venous catheter

PULMONARY EMBOLISM
- Ventilation perfusion scan
- Heparin anticoagulation
- Pulmonary embolectomy

FAT EMBOLISM
- Administration of albumin

AMNIOTIC FLUID EMBOLISM
- "A-OK" medication protocol:
  - Atropine 1 mg IV bolus
  - Ondansetron 8 mg IV bolus
  - Ketorolac 30 mg IV bolus
- Obtain coagulation panel
- Type and crossmatch for packed red blood cells, fresh frozen plasma, and platelets
- Consider uterotonic agents if uterine atony is present

MEDICATIONS
- Vasopressor(s) to maintain MAP > 65 mm Hg:
  - Ephedrine 5 to 10 mg IV bolus and/or,

- Phenylephrine 50 to 100 mcg IV bolus, 0.1 to 0.5 mcg/kg/min infusion and/or,
- Epinephrine 10 to 100 mcg IV bolus, 0.1 to 0.5 mcg/kg/min infusion and/or,
- Dopamine 5 to 20 mcg/kg/min IV infusion and/or,
- Norepinephrine 5 to 10 mcg bolus, 0.1 to 0.5 mcg/kg/min infusion and/or,
- Vasopressin 1 to 4 Unit bolus, 0.01 to 0.1 Units/min infusion

PHYSIOLOGY AND PATHOPHYSIOLOGY

Physiologic manifestations and specific causes of an embolism are presented in Table 14-1. An embolic event results in inadequate

Table 14-1 Signs, symptoms, and causative factors for various types of emboli

	SPECIFIC SIGNS AND SYMPTOMS	CAUSATIVE FACTORS
Air or CO_2 (Gas)	Mill wheel murmur Bubbles in the heart on transesophageal echocardiography **Air embolism:** end-tidal nitrogen on mass spectrometry **CO_2 embolism:** subcutaneous emphysema	**Air embolism:** any procedure when an open vein is positioned above the level of the heart **CO_2 embolism:** occurs during laparoscopic procedures
Amniotic	Bleeding Disseminated intravascular coagulation	Associated with labor and delivery
Pulmonary	Hemoptysis	Associated with DVT Diagnosis-ventilation perfusion scan
Fat	Petechiae Disseminated intravascular coagulation Anemia Low platelets Cor pulmonale	Associated with pelvic and long bone fractures

blood flow through the heart and pulmonary vasculature. The inherent decrease in intracardiac and pulmonary blood flow causes: (1) an increased dead space, (2) ventilation/perfusion mismatch, (3) hypoxemia/hypercarbia, and (4) decreased stroke volume.

1. **Venous air embolism (VAE)** is caused when ambient air is entrained into an open vein. Entrainment most commonly occurs when the surgical site is positioned above the level of the heart (e.g., sitting craniotomy/laminectomy). An airlock is formed as gas congregates at the inflow track to the right atrium. Air can also migrate into the pulmonary artery, causing a right outflow tract obstruction that will further decrease blood flow to the left side of the heart. The result is decreased or absent cardiac output and increased dead space ventilation. The severity of the VAE is determined by the amount of air entrained and the rate of entry.

2. **Carbon dioxide gas embolism** can occur when CO_2 gas used for insufflation during laparoscopic procedures is entrained rapidly and in significant amounts into the central circulation. The remaining pathophysiology is the same as the description for VAE.

3. **Pulmonary embolism** results when an obstruction within the pulmonary artery (e.g., thrombus) impedes pulmonary perfusion and increases dead space. This can cause hypoxemia, decreased stroke volume, and cardiac arrest.

4. **Fat embolism** is frequently associated with pelvic and long bone fractures during trauma. Fat emboli can migrate into lacerated veins and systemic circulation when venous pressure is low, causing cerebrovascular and/or pulmonary artery obstruction. However, fat embolus syndrome can occur during routine surgical procedures such as hip replacement. It is further theorized that as the fat emboli are broken down in the lungs, free fatty acids are released, which can cause interstitial hemorrhaging and pneumocyte dysfunction. The remaining pathophysiology is the same as the description for pulmonary embolism.

5. **Amniotic fluid embolism** is associated with a complex pathophysiologic process. It has been theorized that amniotic fluid, which under normal conditions does not enter maternal circulation, leeches into the bloodstream through endocervical veins at the placental insertion or through a laceration at a site where the uterus has been traumatized.

Pathophysiologic changes associated with AFE occur in two phases.

Phase 1: Severe pulmonary artery vasoconstriction resulting in decreased pulmonary blood flow and hypoxemia, elevated right-sided heart pressure, decreased left ventricular preload, decreased stroke volume, and potential cardiovascular collapse.

Phase 2: Inflammatory mediator release, hemorrhage from uterine atony, and disseminated intravascular coagulation.

SIGNS AND SYMPTOMS (GENERIC TO ALL TYPES OF EMBOLI)

Respiratory

- Decreased/absence of end-tidal carbon dioxide
- Hypercarbia
- Hypoxemia
- Rales/wheezing
- Respiratory arrest
- Shortness of breath
- Tachypnea
- Hemoptysis

Cardiovascular

- Cardiac arrest
- Cardiac dysrhythmias
- Chest pain
- Increased central venous pressure
- Increased pulmonary artery pressure
- Jugular venous distention
- Loss of consciousness
- Tachycardia
- See Table 14-1 for specific signs, symptoms, and causative factors associated with various embolic states

DIFFERENTIAL DIAGNOSIS (GENERIC TO ALL TYPES OF EMBOLI)

Respiratory

- Bronchospasm
- Endotracheal tube obstruction (e.g., mucus plug, kink)
- Hypercarbia
- Hypoxia
- Acute respiratory failure

Cardiovascular

- Acute atrioventricular valvular dysfunction
- Cardiac dysrhythmias
- Cardiogenic shock
- Hypotension
- Myocardial ischemia/infarction

Gastrointestinal

• Acute gastric aspiration

Other considerations

• Anaphylaxis

Diagnostic tests

• Electrocardiogram (ST elevation in lead AVR, S waves in lead I, Q waves/inverted T waves in lead III)
• Computed tomography (pulmonary angiography or ventilation-perfusion scan)
• D-dimer (elevated)
• Chest X-ray
• Coproporphyrin > 35 nmol/L (specific for amniotic fluid embolism)

Suggested Readings

• Brown MH, Darvall J, Hammerschlag G. Acute pulmonary embolism: a concise review of diagnosis and management. *Intern Med J.* 2019;49(1):15-27.
• Elisha S. Posterior reconstructive surgery. In: Elisha S, ed. *Case Studies in Nurse Anesthesia.* St. Louis: Elsevier; 2022:327-338.
• Huffman JS, Humston C, Tobias J. Fat embolism syndrome revisited: a case report and review of literature, with new recommendations for the anesthetized patient. *AANA J.* 2020;88(3):222-228.
• Ranalli LJ, Taylor GA. Obstetric anesthesia. In: Elisha S, Heiner JS, Nagelhout JJ, eds. *Nurse Anesthesia.* 7th ed. St. Louis: Elsevier; 2023:1176-1206.
• Rezai S, Hughes, AC, Larsen TB, Fuller PN, Henderson CE. Atypical amniotic fluid embolism managed with a novel therapeutic regimen. *Case Rep Obstet Gynecol.* 2017;2017: 8458375. doi:10.1155/2017/8458375.

CHAPTER 15   Hypertension

MANAGEMENT

PRIMARY ACTIONS

- Assess noninvasive blood pressure (e.g., inspect blood pressure cuff placement/connection and recheck measurement)
- Assess invasive blood pressure (e.g., confirm appropriate transducer level, ensure the transducer has been zeroed, and perform a fast-flush square-wave test)
- Assess and treat potential causes of severe hypertension
- Increase anesthetic depth
- Provide adequate analgesia
- Administer antihypertensive medications (see "Medications")

SECONDARY ACTIONS

- Arterial line placement as needed

MEDICATIONS

Vasodilators

- Nitroglycerin 5 to 10 mcg IV bolus, 5 to 100 mcg/min IV infusion and/or,
- Nitroprusside 0.2 to 0.5 mcg/kg/min IV infusion and/or,
- Hydralazine 5 mg IV bolus every 10 minutes, up to 20 mg total dose and/or,
- Clevidipine 1 to 20 mg/h IV infusion and/or,

Beta-blockers

- Esmolol 0.5 to 1 mg/kg IV bolus, 0.15 to 0.3 mg/kg/min IV infusion and/or,
- Labetalol 5 mg IV bolus every 5 minutes, up to 50 mg total dose and/or,

Calcium channel blocker

- Nicardipine 0.2 to 0.5 mg IV bolus, 2.5 to 15 mg/h infusion

PHYSIOLOGY AND PATHOPHYSIOLOGY

Arterial autoregulation is the ability of arteries to dilate and constrict over a range of blood pressures to maintain a constant blood flow. In humans, coronary and cerebral artery autoregulation occurs between mean arterial pressure values of 60 to 140 mm Hg. Above the autoregulatory limits, coronary and cerebral blood flow becomes pressure-dependent. These high pressures can cause acute myocardial ischemia/infarction, hemorrhagic cerebrovascular accident, or congestive heart failure.

Severe hypertension and increased systemic vascular resistance increase myocardial workload and oxygen demand. This can result

Table 15-1 Classification of hypertension for adults age 18 years and older

CATEGORY	
Normal	$< 120/ < 80$ mm Hg
Elevated	$120\text{-}129 / < 80$ mm Hg
Hypertension stage 1	SBP 130-139 or DBP 80-89
Hypertension stage 2	SBP $\geq$ 140 or DBP $\geq$ 90

Abbreviations: DBP, diastolic blood pressure; SBP, systolic blood pressure

in decreased stroke volume, cardiac output, congestive heart failure, and/or shock. Furthermore, severe untreated perioperative hypertension can result in bleeding from the operative site. The National Institutes of Health have created a classification system based on the degree of hypertension (Table 15-1). Untreated, prolonged (chronic) hypertension contributes to vascular pathology that can result in: (1) atherosclerosis, (2) renal dysfunction/failure, (3) aortic and cerebral aneurysms, (4) myocardial hypertrophy, (5) myocardial infarction, (6) hemorrhagic cerebrovascular accident, and (7) congestive heart failure.

SIGNS AND SYMPTOMS

Neurologic

- Altered level of consciousness
- Anxiety
- Blurred vision
- Headache
- Hemorrhagic stroke
- Papilledema

Respiratory

- Shortness of breath
- Tachypnea

Cardiovascular

- Bounding peripheral pulses
- Congestive heart failure
- Dysrhythmias
- Increased pulse pressure
- Increased systolic/diastolic blood pressure
- Myocardial ischemia/infarction

Renal

- Decreased renal function
- Proteinuria

Other considerations

- Epistaxis

DIFFERENTIAL DIAGNOSIS

Neurologic

- Autonomic hyperreflexia
- Increased intracranial pressure (Cushing's triad)

Respiratory

- Airway obstruction
- Hypercarbia
- Hypoxia

Cardiovascular

- Fluid overload
- Primary (essential) hypertension
- Renovascular hypertension
- Surgical compression of major vasculature (e.g., aortic cross-clamp placement)
- Sympathetic nervous system stimulation
  1. Surgical stimulation
  2. Inadequate depth of anesthesia
  3. Intubation
  4. Stimulation of the carina by endotracheal tube
  5. Emergence

Endocrine

- Cushing syndrome
- Pheochromocytoma
- Thyrotoxicosis

Pharmacologic

- Adrenergic agonists (e.g., vasopressors, ketamine)
- Drug withdrawal
- Malignant hyperthermia
- Medication error
- Naloxone
- Omission of prescribed antihypertensive medications
- Sympathomimetic drug misuse (e.g., cocaine, methamphetamine)
- Vasopressor medications

Other considerations

- Anxiety
- Distended bladder
- Equipment problem
    1. Arterial catheter-line transducer inappropriately positioned below the level of the heart
    2. External pressure on the blood pressure cuff by the surgical staff
    3. Blood pressure cuff that is too small for the patient's arm
- Hypoglycemia
- Malignant hyperthermia
- Pain
- Preeclampsia/eclampsia

Diagnostic tests

- Blood urea nitrogen/creatinine, glomerular filtration rate
- Chest X-ray
- Echocardiography
- Electrocardiogram
- Preoperative cardiac workup and clearance

Suggested Readings

- Elisha S. Cardiovascular anatomy, physiology, pathophysiology, and anesthesia management. In: Elisha S, Heiner JS, Nagelhout JJ, eds. *Nurse Anesthesia.* 7th ed. St. Louis: Elsevier; 2023:477-515.
- Howell SJ. Preoperative hypertension. *Curr Anesthesiol Rep.* 2018;8(1):25-31.
- McEvoy MD, Gupta R, Koepke EJ, et al. Perioperative Quality Initiative consensus statement on postoperative blood pressure, risk and outcomes for elective surgery. *Br J Anaesth.* 2019;122(5):575-586.
- Watson K, Broscious R, Devabhakthuni S, Noel ZR. Focused update on pharmacologic management of hypertensive emergencies. *Curr Hypertens Rep.* 2018;20(7):56.
- Whelton PK, Carey RM, Aronow WS, et al. 2017 ACC/AHA/AAPA/ABC/ACPM/AGS/APhA/ASH/ASPC/NMA/PCNA guideline for the prevention, detection, evaluation, and management of high blood pressure in adults: a report of the American College of Cardiology/American Heart Association Task Force on Clinical Practice Guidelines. *J Am Coll Cardiol.* 2018;71:e127-e248.

CHAPTER 16 Hypotension

MANAGEMENT

PRIMARY ACTIONS
- Assess *noninvasive* blood pressure (e.g., appropriately sized cuff, placementt/connection, external compression, and recheck measurement)
- Assess invasive blood pressure (e.g., confirm transducer level, ensure the transducer has been zeroed to atmospheric pressure, and perform a fast-flush with square-wave test)
- Administer FiO_2 to maintain oxygen saturation $> 90\%$
- Decrease or discontinue administration of anesthetic agents
- Identify and treat the cause of severe hypotension
- Insert second peripheral intravenous and/or central venous catheter
- Expand intravascular volume
  1. Crystalloids
  2. Colloids (albumin)
  3. Packed red blood cells, fresh frozen plasma, and platelets if hemorrhage/anemia is present
- Elevate lower extremities and/or place in slight Trendelenburg position
- Maintain a secure and patent airway
- Minimize peak inspiratory pressure and positive end-expiratory pressure

SECONDARY ACTIONS
- Arterial line placement and monitoring as needed
- Confirm that a rapid infuser is available
- Obtain laboratory analysis as needed (e.g., hemoglobin/hematocrit, electrolytes, glucose)
- Arterial blood gas

MEDICATIONS
- Vasopressor(s) to maintain mean arterial pressure (MAP) > 65 mm Hg:
  - Ephedrine 5 to 10 mg IV bolus and/or,
  - Phenylephrine 50 to 100 mcg IV bolus, 0.1 to 0.5 mcg/kg/min infusion and/or,
  - Epinephrine 10 to 100 mcg IV bolus, 0.1 to 0.5 mcg/kg/min infusion and/or,
  - Dopamine 5 to 20 mcg/kg/min IV infusion and/or,
  - Norepinephrine 5 to 10 mcg bolus, 0.1 to 0.5 mcg/kg/min infusion and/or,
  - Vasopressin 1 to 4 Unit bolus, 0.01 to 0.1 Units/min infusion
  - Methylene blue 1 to 2 mg/kg over 20 to 60 minutes, 0.5 to 1 mg/kg/h infusion

PHYSIOLOGY AND PATHOPHYSIOLOGY

A universally accepted definition for hypotension does not exist. Several guidelines have been suggested in an attempt to quantify intraoperative hypotension: (1) systolic blood pressure < 90 mm Hg, (2) diastolic blood pressure < 60 mm Hg, (3) MAP < 60 mm Hg, and (4) greater than a 20% decrease in blood pressure compared with preoperative values.

The most significant concern associated with severe and sustained hypotension includes end-organ (e.g., cerebral and/or myocardial) ischemia. Arterial autoregulation is the ability of arteries to dilate and constrict over a range of blood pressures to maintain a constant blood flow. In humans, coronary and cerebral artery autoregulation occurs between MAP readings of 60 and 140 mm Hg. Below the autoregulatory limits, cerebral and coronary blood flow becomes pressure-dependent (pressure-passive). Furthermore, patients with cerebral and/or coronary artery pathology (e.g., plaque lesions) may require a higher MAP to maintain adequate perfusion.

Vasoplegic syndrome (paralysis of the vasculature) can result in hypotension refractory to the most common initial interventions. It is caused by an increase in inducible nitric oxide, which is a potent vasodilator. Vasopressor medications that are adrenergic agonists may not adequately treat refractory hypotension. Alternative pharmacologic agents such as vasopressin and methylene blue can help treat hypotension if vasoplegic syndrome exists.

SIGNS AND SYMPTOMS

Neurologic
- Altered level of consciousness
- Cerebral ischemia
- Ischemia stroke
- Nausea/vomiting

Respiratory
- Airway obstruction-late sign
- Shortness of breath

Cardiovascular
- Cardiac arrest
- Chest pain
- Decreased EtCO$_2$
- Decreased peripheral/central pulses
- Decreased systolic/diastolic blood pressure
- Dysrhythmias
- Low and or narrowed pulse pressure

- Prolonged capillary refill/pale skin
- Tachycardia

Renal

- Metabolic acidosis
- Oliguria

DIFFERENTIAL DIAGNOSIS

Respiratory

- Hypoxia (late sign)
- Positive end-expiratory pressure
- Tension pneumothorax

Cardiovascular

- Acute cardiac valve insufficiency
- All shock states
- Cardiac dysrhythmias
- Excessive abdominal pressure caused by pneumoperitoneum during laparoscopic surgery
- Hypertrophic cardiomyopathy
- Hypovolemia
- Increased insufflation pressures during laparoscopic surgery
- Myocardial ischemia/infarction
- Parasympathetic nervous system predominance
- Pressure by the surgeon on major vascular structures
- Reflex bradycardia/vasodilation (e.g., celiac, oculocardiac, Bezold-Jarisch reflex)
- Reperfusion of ischemic tissue (e.g., removal of the aortic cross-clamp)
- Valvular heart disease

Endocrine

- Acute adrenal crises
- Hypothyroidism
- Period immediately following venous ligation during adrenal-ectomy for pheochromocytoma

Hematologic

- Anemia
- Hemorrhage

Pharmacologic

- Anesthetic induction agents/inhalation agents
- Continuation of preoperative angiotensin-converting enzyme inhibitor/angiotensin receptor blocker and or diuretics
- Excessive beta blockade or calcium channel blockade

- Histamine release (e.g., atracurium)
- Inhalation agents
- Local anesthetic toxicity
- Medication error
- Narcotics
- Neuraxial anesthesia
- Reversal of heparin with protamine
- Total spinal anesthetic
- Vasodilating agents

Other considerations

- Anaphylaxis
- Assessment error/artifact
  1. Arterial catheter transducer inappropriately positioned above the heart
  2. External pressure on the blood pressure cuff by the surgical staff
  3. Inappropriately sized blood pressure cuff that is typically too large
- Embolism (e.g., thrombus, air, fat)
- Hypermagnesemia
- Hypocalcemia
- Hypoglycemia (rapid onset in neonates)
- Pregnancy (e.g., aortocaval compression)

Diagnostic tests

- Electrocardiogram
- Laboratory tests: hemoglobin/hematocrit, electrolytes, glucose
- Ultrasound assessment of inferior vena cava collapsibility

Suggested Readings

- Chaix I, Manquat E, Liu N, et al. Impact of hypotension on cerebral perfusion during general anesthesia induction: a prospective observational study in adults. *Acta Anaesthesiol Scand.* 2020;64(5):592-601.
- Elisha S. Cardiovascular anatomy, physiology, pathophysiology, and anesthesia management. In: Elisha S, Heiner JS, Nagelhout JJ, eds. *Nurse Anesthesia.* 7th ed. St. Louis: Elsevier; 2023:477-515.
- Hallqvist L, Granath F, Fored M, Bell M. Intraoperative hypotension and myocardial infarction development among high-risk patients undergoing noncardiac surgery: a nested case-control study. *Anesth Analg.* 2021;133(1):6-15.
- Sessler DI, Bloomstone JA, Aronson S, et al. Perioperative Quality Initiative consensus statement on intraoperative blood pressure, risk and outcomes for elective surgery. *Br J Anaesth.* 2019;122(5):563-574.

CHAPTER 17   Myocardial Ischemia and Infarction

PRIMARY ACTIONS

- Inform the surgeon and complete the surgical procedure
- Monitor and support airway, breathing, and circulation
- Confirm diagnosis
  1. See "Signs and Symptoms"
  2. Obtain 12-lead electrocardiogram
  3. Transesophageal or transthoracic echocardiography
  4. Obtain cardiac enzymes (troponin and creatine kinase-MB)
- Pharmacologic treatment (see "Medications" and Table 17-1)
- Cardiology consultation
- Invasive monitoring (e.g., arterial line)

SECONDARY ACTIONS

- Consult American Heart Association management for acute coronary syndrome
- Perform ACLS or PALS per American Heart Association protocol
- Prepare for a higher level of cardiac intensive care
  1. Cardiac catheterization
  2. Anticoagulation (aspirin and/or heparin)
  3. Fibrinolytic therapy

MEDICATIONS

- Vasodilators
  - Nitroglycerin 5 to 10 mcg IV bolus, 5 to 100 mcg/min IV infusion and/or,
  - Nitroprusside 0.2 to 0.5 mcg/kg/min IV infusion and/or,
  - Hydralazine 5 mg IV bolus every 10 minutes, up to 20 mg total dose and/or,
  - Clevidipine 1 to 20 mg/h IV infusion
- Beta blockers
  - Esmolol 0.5 to 1 mg/kg IV bolus, 0.15 to 0.3 mg/kg/min IV infusion and/or,
  - Labetalol 5 mg IV bolus every 5 minutes, up to 50 mg total dose and/or,
- Calcium channel blocker
  - Nicardipine 0.2 to 0.5 mg IV bolus, 2.5 to 15 mg/h infusion
- Vasopressor(s) to maintain mean arterial pressure > 65 mm Hg:
  - Ephedrine 5 to 10 mg IV bolus and/or,
  - Phenylephrine 50 to 100 mcg IV bolus, 0.1 to 0.5 mcg/kg/min infusion and/or,
  - Epinephrine 10 to 100 mcg IV bolus, 0.1 to 0.5 mcg/kg/min infusion and/or,

- Dopamine 5 to 20 mcg/kg/min IV infusion and/or,
- Norepinephrine 5 to 10 mcg bolus, 0.1 to 0.5 mcg/kg/min infusion and/or,
- Vasopressin 1 to 4 Unit bolus, 0.01 to 0.1 Units/min infusion

Table 17-1 Treatment for intraoperative myocardial ischemia/infarction

HEMODYNAMIC EVENT	THERAPY	PHARMACOLOGIC GOALS
Hypertension/ tachycardia	• Increase anesthetic depth • IV beta blockade, and/or • IV nitroglycerin	• ↓SNS reactivity • ↓inotropy/chronotropy • ↓preload/wall tension, dilates epicardial vessels
Normotensive/ tachycardia	• Confirm adequate anesthetic depth • IV beta blockade	• ↓SNS reactivity • ↓inotropy/chronotropy
Hypertension/ normal HR	• Increase anesthetic depth • IV nitroglycerin or nicardipine	• ↓SVR, myocardial depression • ↓preload/wall tension, dilates epicardial vessels
Hypotension/ tachycardia	• IV fluid bolus • Decrease anesthetic depth • IV Phenylephrine • IV nitroglycerin when normotensive	• ↑intravascular volume • ↑systemic vascular resistance • ↓preload/wall tension, dilates epicardial vessels
Hypotension/ bradycardia	• Ensure oxygenation • Decrease anesthetic depth • IV ephedrine, and/or • IV epinephrine, and/or • IV atropine, and/or • IV nitroglycerin when normotensive	• Eliminate hypoxia at the cardioaccelerator center • ↑systemic vascular resistance • ↑inotropy/chronotropy • ↓PNS reactivity • ↓preload/wall tension, dilates epicardial vessels

Table 17-1 Treatment for intraoperative myocardial ischemia/ infarction—cont'd

HEMODYNAMIC EVENT	THERAPY	PHARMACOLOGIC GOALS
Hypotension/ normal HR	• Decrease anesthetic depth • IV phenylephrine, and/or • IV ephedrine, and/or • IV epinephrine, and/or • IV nitroglycerin when normotensive	• ↑systemic vascular resistance • ↑inotropy/chronotropy • ↓preload/wall tension, dilates epicardial vessels
Ischemia/infarction without hemodynamic abnormality	• IV nitroglycerin and/or • IV nicardipine	• ↓preload/wall tension, ilates epicardial vessels

Abbreviations: HR, heart rate; PNS, parasympathetic nervous system; SNS, sympathetic nervous system; SVR, systemic vascular resistance.

PHYSIOLOGY AND PATHOPHYSIOLOGY

During anesthesia and surgery, physiologic stress causes hemodynamic variability throughout the perioperative process. Factors that increase myocardial oxygen demand in relation to supply predispose the myocardium to ischemia and infarction. Factors that influence myocardial supply and demand are listed in Table 17-2. Increased heart rate is pertinent in both the demand (e.g., increased cellular energy utilized) and supply (e.g., decreased diastolic perfusion time for the left ventricle) sides of the myocardial oxygen balance. Thus, heart rate is the factor that, when increased, decreases myocardial oxygenation to the greatest degree. When myocardial oxygen deprivation occurs, myocardial excitation-contraction

Table 17-2 Factors that influence myocardial oxygen supply and demand

SUPPLY	DEMAND
• Decreased heart rate	• Increased heart rate
• Coronary blood flow	• Preload
• Diastolic blood pressure	• Afterload
• Oxygenated hemoglobin	• Contractility

coupling is inhibited because of a lack of adenosine triphosphate production. Cardiac wall motion abnormalities ensue and, if untreated, cardiogenic shock can occur. Rapid diagnosis and treatment are essential to inhibit myocardial damage and preserve myocardial function. Acute electrocardiogram changes, dysrhythmias, and hypotension are classic signs of cardiac ischemia or infarction. Treatment strategies for management are included in Table 17-1. Perioperative myocardial infarction is associated with a significantly increased incidence of postoperative mortality.

SIGNS AND SYMPTOMS

Neurologic

- Altered/loss of consciousness
- Dizziness
- Syncope

Respiratory

- Hypercarbia
- Hypoxia
- Rales
- Respiratory arrest
- Shortness of breath
- Tachypnea

Cardiovascular

- Cardiac arrest
- Cardiogenic shock
- Chest pain with or without radiation
- Congestive heart failure
- Decreased capillary refill
- Decreased ejection fraction
- Decreased peripheral pulses
- Diaphoresis
- Electrocardiogram
  1. Dysrhythmias
  2. New-onset atrioventricular or bundle branch block
  3. New-onset T-wave inversion
  4. ST-segment elevation/depression
- Elevated cardiac troponin and creatine kinase-MB
- Hemodynamic profile
  1. Hypertension/hypotension
  2. Increased central venous pressure
  3. Increased pulmonary capillary wedge pressure
  4. Increased systemic vascular resistance
  5. Tachycardia/bradycardia

- New-onset cardiac murmur
- Pain to the jaw and or left arm
- Ventricular wall motion abnormalities on transesophageal echocardiography

DIFFERENTIAL DIAGNOSIS

Neurologic

- Anxiety
- Cerebrovascular accident

Respiratory

- Pleuritis
- Pulmonary embolism

Cardiovascular

- Acute aortic dissection
- Cardiac tamponade
- Coronary artery vasospasm
- Costochondritis
- Pericarditis
- Shock states

Gastrointestinal

- Dyspepsia/gastroesophageal reflux disease

Other considerations

- Acute adrenal crises
- Anaphylaxis
- Cholecystitis
- Intercostal muscle spasm
- Pancreatitis
- Trauma (e.g., cardiac contusion)

Suggested Readings

- Cormican DS, Sonny A, Crowley J, et al. Acute myocardial infarction complicated by cardiogenic shock: analysis of the position statement from the European Society of Cardiology Acute Cardiovascular Care Association, with perioperative implications. *J Cardiothorac Vasc Anesth*. 2021;35(10):3098-3104.
- Elisha S. Cardiovascular anatomy, physiology, pathophysiology, and anesthesia management. In: Elisha S, Heiner JS, Nagelhout JJ, eds. *Nurse Anesthesia*. 7th ed. St. Louis: Elsevier; 2023:477-515.

- Hallqvist L, Granath F, Fored M, Bell M. Intraoperative hypotension and myocardial infarction development among high-risk patients undergoing noncardiac surgery: a nested case-control study. *Anesth Analg.* 2021;133(1):6-15.
- Samsky MD, Morrow DA, Proudfoot AG, Hochman JS, Thiele H, Rao SV. Cardiogenic shock after acute myocardial infarction: a review. *JAMA.* 2021;326(18):1840-1850.
- Smilowitz NR, Berger JS. Perioperative cardiovascular risk assessment and management for noncardiac surgery: a review. *JAMA.* 2020;324(3):279-290.
- Smit M, Coetzee AR, Lochner A. The pathophysiology of myocardial ischemia and perioperative myocardial infarction. *J Cardiothorac Vasc Anesth.* 2020;34(9):2501-2512.

CHAPTER 18 Pacemakers and Automated Internal Cardiac Defibrillators (AICDs)

MANAGEMENT

PRIMARY ACTIONS

- Determine if the cardiac implantable electronic device (CIED) is a cardiac pacemaker and/or automatic implantable cardioverter-defibrillator (AICD)
- Determine the manufacturer, primary indication for placement, current settings, and if the patient is pacer-dependent
- Continuously monitor cardiac rate, rhythm, and peripheral pulses
- Ensure that temporary pacing and defibrillation equipment are immediately available
- If electromagnetic interference is likely to occur (e.g., electrocautery near CIED), place a magnet over the CIED to:
  1. Alter the pacing function to an asynchronous pacing mode in pacemaker-dependent patients
  2. Suspend a CIED's active sensor for rate-responsive pacing to prevent undesirable tachycardia
  3. Suspend an AICD's antitachycardia function

SECONDARY ACTIONS

- Minimize the risk of electromagnetic interference (EMI) from monopolar electrosurgery
  1. Position the electrosurgical instrument and grounding pad, so the electrical current pathway does not pass through or near the CIED or intracardiac leads
  2. Use short and intermittent bursts of electrosurgery at the lowest energy levels necessary
  3. Use bipolar electrosurgery or an ultrasonic (harmonic) scalpel
- For emergency pacing, cardioversion, or defibrillation:
  1. Terminate all sources of EMI
  2. Remove the magnet to restore the CIED function
  3. If the CIED function is unrestored, institute current ACLS/PALS guidelines
- Consultation with a cardiologist or manufacturer to interrogate, restore, or reprogram the CIED settings

PHYSIOLOGY/PATHOPHYSIOLOGY

During a normal cardiac cycle, the heart's conduction pathways and structural components work in coordination to produce a heartbeat. This synchrony is vital for blood oxygenation and cardiac output, and ultimately adequate oxygen delivery to peripheral and central tissues. Cardiac dysrhythmias represent conduction and/or structural abnormalities of the cardiac cycle. Medical management of cardiac bradyarrhythmias, tachyarrhythmias, or heart failure may include placing a CEID (e.g., cardiac pacemaker, AICD).

Safe and effective perioperative management of a CIED is imperative to minimize adverse outcomes such as (1) device or lead-tissue interface damage; (2) failure of device to pace or deliver shocks; (3) pacing or shock delivery when not indicated; and (4) alterations in pacing behavior or reset to backup pacing mode. EMI may be misinterpreted as intracardiac impulses by a CIED device, giving rise to abnormal behavior and potentially severe adverse outcomes. Potential sources of EMI include:
- electrocautery
- radiofrequency ablation
- lithotripsy
- magnetic resonance imaging
- radiation therapy
- radiofrequency identification devices
- electroconvulsive therapy

SIGNS AND SYMPTOMS

Neurologic
- Altered level of consciousness
- Syncope

Respiratory
- Dyspnea
- Hypercarbia
- Hypoxemia
- Tachypnea

Cardiovascular
- Cardiac dysrhythmias
- Hypotension
- Left ventricular dysfunction
- Loss of central and/or peripheral pulses
- Myocardial infarction or ischemia

- Myocardial lead-tissue damage
- Right- or left-sided heart failure

DIFFERENTIAL DIAGNOSIS

Neurologic

- Ischemic stroke

Respiratory

- Pulmonary edema
- Pulmonary embolus

Cardiovascular

- Conduction cardiac disease
    1. First-, second-, or third-degree atrioventricular nodal block
    2. Brugada syndrome
    3. Fascicular or bundle branch block
    4. Q-T interval prolongation
    5. Sinus bradycardia (e.g., hemodynamic compromise)
    6. Sinus node dysfunction (e.g., sick sinus syndrome)
    7. Supraventricular tachycardia
    8. Torsades de pointes
    9. Ventricular fibrillation
    10. Ventricular tachycardia
    11. Wolff-Parkinson-White syndrome
- Structural cardiac disease
    1. Cardiomyopathy (e.g., concentric or eccentric)
    2. Cardiopulmonary disease (e.g., chronic obstructive pulmonary disease)
    3. Congenital cardiac disease
    4. Coronary artery disease
    5. Inflammatory disease (e.g., pericarditis)
    6. Postcardiac surgical intervention
    7. Right- or left-sided heart failure
    8. Valvular cardiac disease

Suggested Reading

- American Society of Anesthesiologists Task Force on Perioperative Management of Patients with Cardiac Implantable Electronic Devices. Practice advisory for the perioperative management of patients with cardiac implantable electronic devices: pacemakers and implantable cardioverter-defibrillators. *Anesthesiology.* 2020;132(2):225-252.

- Ashlock BJ, Franco JA. Perioperative management for patients with cardiac devices. In: Elisha S, Heiner JS, Nagelhout JJ, eds. *Nurse Anesthesia*. 7th ed. St. Louis: Elsevier; 2023:574-585.
- Mattingly E. Arrhythmia management devices and electromagnetic interference. *AANA J*. 2005;73(2):129-136.
- Ray SB, Poepsel A. Anesthetic management of a laboring patient with a closed-loop stimulation pacemaker: a case report. *AANA J*. 2019;87(6):483-488.

CHAPTER 19   Acute Cerebral Vascular Accident

MANAGEMENT

PRIMARY ACTIONS

- Increase FiO_2 to 100%
- Initiate specialized stroke protocols and mobilize Stroke Team if available
- Primary anesthetic goals:
  1. Minimize time to revascularization
  2. Hemodynamic control
- Arrange consultation with neurologist and perform stroke severity assessment
- Evaluate blood glucose level
- Noncontrast computerized tomography scan (as soon as possible on arrival)
- Confirm two large bore IVs
- Consider intubation if the patient cannot protect the airway
  - Avoid hypoxia, hypercarbia, or hypocarbia
- Place arterial line
  - Maintain arterial blood pressure within 20% of baseline value (keep systolic blood pressure [SBP] > 110 mm Hg)
  - American Heart Association recommends BP < 185/110 for patients with hypertension
- Support revascularization during ischemic stroke:
  - IV treatment with tPA (alteplase) if criteria is met and within 3-4.5 hours of initial symptoms (see "Medications")
  - Expedite endovascular therapy within 6 to 24 hours after initial symptoms
- Maintain mean arterial pressure (MAP) > 70 mm Hg during intraprocedural endovascular mechanical thrombectomy
- After revascularization, maintain a MAP > 70 mm Hg. Goal is to keep SBP:
  - < 180 mm Hg after IV tPA treatment
  - < 160 mm Hg after mechanical thrombectomy
  - < 140 mm Hg for an intracerebral hemorrhagic lesion

SECONDARY ACTIONS

- Avoid and treat hyperthermia
- Transfuse if hemoglobin levels < 8 g/dL

- If providing general anesthesia for endovascular therapy, prepare vasopressor and antihypertensive agents (see "Medications")
  - Avoid using metoprolol to manage hypertension
- Ventilate using lung protective strategy (Vt 6-8 mL/kg and keep plateau pressures < 30 mm Hg)
- General anesthesia (GA) or sedation with local anesthesia for endovascular mechanical thrombectomy (see Table 19-1)
- GA recommended for endovascular recanalization in patients with:
  - Agitation
  - Reduced Glasgow Coma Scale
  - Nausea and vomiting
  - Large dominant hemisphere stroke
  - Posterior circulation stroke

MEDICATIONS

- Vasopressor(s) to maintain MAP > 70 mm Hg:
  - Ephedrine 5-10 mg IV bolus and/or,
  - Phenylephrine 50-100 mcg IV bolus, 0.1-0.5 mcg/kg/min infusion and/or,
  - Epinephrine 10-100 mcg IV bolus, 0.1-0.5 mcg/kg/min infusion and/or,
  - Norepinephrine 5-10 mcg IV bolus, 0.1-0.5 mcg/kg/min infusion and/or,
  - Vasopressin 1-2 Unit IV bolus, 0.01-0.05 Units/min infusion

Table 19-1 Comparison of Anesthetic Technique for Endovascular Therapy After Acute CVA

GENERAL ANESTHESIA	SEDATION WITH LOCAL ANESTHESIA
Advantages	*Advantages*
Immobility that reduces the risk of vascular injury	Hemodynamic stability
Airway protection	Ability to evaluate neurological status
Pain and anxiety control	Less risk of respiratory depression
	Rapid time to procedure
Disadvantages	*Disadvantages*
Potential hemodynamic instability	No airway protection and potential for aspiration
Potential for respiratory depression	Patient movement during procedure
Potential for aspiration	Uncontrolled pain and agitation
Delay to start of procedure	

- Antihypertensive agents:
  - Esmolol 10 mg IV bolus (titrate to effect) or,
  - Labetalol 10-20 mg IV bolus over 2 minutes and/or,
  - Nicardipine 5 mg/h IV infusion (can increase 2.5 mg/h every 5-15 minutes up to maximum dose of 15 mg/h) or,
  - Clevidipine 1-2 mg/h IV infusion (can increase 1-2 mg/h every 2-5 minutes up to maximum dose of 21 mg/h) and/or,
  - Sodium nitroprusside 0.3-0.5 mcg/kg/min (up to 2 mcg/kg/min) infusion
- Aspirin 81-162 mg PO after thrombectomy within 24-48 hours if no contraindications. Hold for 24 hours if patient received IV tPA.
- tPA (alteplase) 0.9 mg/kg IV. Give 10% of total dose as bolus over 1 minute, then give remaining 90% as IV infusion over 60 minutes. Do not administer more than 90 mg.

PHYSIOLOGY AND PATHOPHYSIOLOGY

An acute cerebral vascular accident (CVA), or "stroke," can be caused by a cerebral artery embolus, thrombus, stenosis, or intracranial hemorrhage. Strokes are more often caused by cerebral ischemia compared with intracranial hemorrhage. Following the initial ischemic insult, reduced perfusion to the ischemic area can occur from (1) cerebrovascular occlusion, (2) cytotoxic edema from the injured brain, and (3) impaired cerebral autoregulation.

An early primary goal is reperfusion of the blocked cerebral vessel. If a patient presents early enough (within 3-4.5 hours of symptom onset), they can be medically treated with IV recombinant tissue plasminogen activator (tPA). Patients who present after the tPA cutoff time, have contraindications to tPA (see Table 19-2), or if tPA has failed may be considered for endovascular therapy using intra-arterial thrombolysis or mechanical clot removal.

The incidence of perioperative stroke after noncardiac surgery is between 0.1% to 1%. Ischemic stroke during anesthesia may result because of (1) decreased perfusion to the brain from significant hypotension, (2) carotid atherosclerotic disease and potential cerebral embolism, or (3) intracranial hemorrhage. Hypotension that reduces cerebral perfusion can occur for a variety of reasons (see Differential Diagnosis section). Atherosclerotic disease of the carotid vessels can occur from subintimal fatty plaques that increase in size over time and eventually occlude the vascular lumen to some degree. This leads to decreased cerebral blood flow and even a risk of plaque rupture causing a cerebral embolus. Intracranial hemorrhage is rare during anesthesia and is usually the result of prior trauma or surgical craniotomy.

Table 19-2 Contraindications to intravenous thrombolytic treatment

- Subarachnoid or intracranial hemorrhage
- Active internal bleeding
- Stroke within last 3 months
- Mass lesions of the brain
- Major surgery within the past 15 days
- Persistent hypertension (systolic blood pressure > 185 mm Hg, diastolic blood pressure > 110 mm Hg)
- History of bleeding or coagulation problems (platelets < 100,000, international normalized ratio > 1.7, and prothrombin time > 15)
- Hypoglycemia (glucose < 50 mg/dL)
- NIHSS < 6

NIHSS, National Institute of Health Stroke Scale

Adequate cerebral perfusion pressure (CPP) should be maintained during acute CVA to promote cerebral blood flow (CBF). Normally, CPP is calculated by subtracting the intracranial pressure (ICP) from the mean arterial pressure (MAP). Autoregulation of CPP (e.g., MAP of 60-160 mm Hg) may be decreased after an acute CVA. Thus, a higher MAP is required to maintain adequate CPP and CBF. In the event the patient presents with perioperative hypertension and symptoms of CVA, efforts to maintain a systolic blood pressure of < 180 mm Hg but > 110 mm Hg should be employed.

Cerebral perfusion pressures can be altered because of factors controlled by anesthesia management, such as carbon dioxide levels and inhalation anesthetic concentrations. Cerebral vascular constriction can happen with profound hypocarbia. In contrast, cerebral steal may occur with hypercarbia causing cerebral vasodilation which can divert blood away from oxygen-starved and damaged brain tissue. Inhalation of anesthetic agents causes cerebral artery vasodilation in a dose-dependent manner and consequently results in an increase in CBF. This can further increase ICP and decrease CPP and CBF.

SIGNS AND SYMPTOMS

Neurologic

- Hallmark of perioperative stroke is the onset of sudden focal neurologic deficits
- Aphasia
- Agitation
- Autonomic instability

- Delayed emergence from anesthesia
- Delirium
- Dysequilibrium
- Dysphagia
- Dizziness
- Facial droop
- Headache
- Hemiparesis
- History of stroke
- Mental status changes
- Sensory deficits
- Seizures
- Vertigo
- Vision disturbances

Respiratory

- Desaturation
- Hypoxemia
- Inability to regain spontaneous ventilation after anesthesia
- Loss of airway reflexes

Cardiovascular

- Hypertension
- Tachycardia
- Arrhythmias

Other considerations

- Temperature dysregulation

DIFFERENTIAL DIAGNOSIS

Neurological

- Bell's palsy
- Brain tumor
- Complex migraine
- Encephalitis
- Multiple sclerosis
- Spinal or epidural hematoma
- Transient ischemic attack

Respiratory

- Refractory hypoxemia

Cardiovascular

- Acute hypertensive crisis
- Autonomic insufficiency

- Significant intraoperative hypotension:
  - Anaphylaxis
  - Cardiogenic shock
  - Cardiac compressive shock
  - Excessive anesthesia medications
  - Hypovolemic or hemorrhagic shock
  - Neurogenic shock
  - Sepsis or septic shock

Endocrine

- Hyperglycemia
- Hypoglycemia

Pharmacologic

- Excessive opioid administration
- Drug misuse (e.g., Sympathomimetics-cocaine, methamphetamines)
- Perioperative use of beta blockers
- Prolonged effects of anesthetic medications (e.g., inhalation agents, propofol, etomidate, ketamine)
- Residual neuromuscular blockade

Other considerations

- Delayed emergence from anesthesia
- Medication error (e.g., administration of high dose phenylephrine or epinephrine)
- Local anesthetic systemic toxicity (LAST)
- Sepsis

Diagnostic tests

- Arterial blood gas
- Computed tomography scan noncontrast
- Computed tomography angiography
- Electrocardiogram
- Electroencephalographic slow wave activity
- Evaluate electrolytes, renal function, and coagulation status
- Hemoglobin and hematocrit
- May consider evaluating neurological biomarkers such as S-100β, neuron-specific enolase, matrix metalloproteinase-9, and glial fibrillary acid protein levels
- Toxicology screen

Suggested Readings

- Benesch C, Glance LG, Derdeyn CP, et al. Perioperative neurological evaluation and management to lower the risk of acute stroke in patients undergoing noncardiac, nonneurological surgery: a scientific statement from the American Heart Association/American Stroke Association. *Circulation*. 2021;143(19):e923-e946.
- Businger J, Fort AC, Vlisides PE, et al. Management of acute ischemic stroke-specific focus on anesthetic management for mechanical thrombectomy. *Anesth Analg*. 2020;131(4):1124-1134.
- Dinsmore J, Elwishi M, Kailainathan P. Anaesthesia for endovascular thrombectomy. *BJA Educ*. 2018;18(10):291-299.
- Elisha S. Anesthesia for vascular surgery. In: Elisha S, Heiner JS, Nagelhout JJ, eds. *Nurse Anesthesia*. 7th ed. St. Louis: Elsevier; 2023:586-613.
- Goyal N, Malhotra K, Ishfaq MF, et al. Current evidence for anesthesia management during endovascular stroke therapy: updated systematic review and meta-analysis. *J Neurointerv Surg*. 2019;11(2):107-113.
- Löwhagen Hendén P, Rentzos A, Karlsson JE, et al. General anesthesia versus conscious sedation for endovascular treatment of acute ischemic stroke: The AnStroke Trial (Anesthesia During Stroke). *Stroke*. 2017;48(6):1601-1607.
- Vitt JR, Trillanes M, Hemphill JC III. Management of blood pressure during and after recanalization therapy for acute ischemic stroke. *Front Neurol*. 2019;10:138.

CHAPTER 20   Increased Intracranial Pressure

MANAGEMENT

PRIMARY ACTIONS

- Maintain CPP = (MAP – ICP)
  - Keep MAP 80-100 mm Hg (except for intracerebral hemorrhage)
  - For intracerebral hemorrhage, maintain systolic blood pressure of 140 mm Hg
- Administer FiO_2 100%
- Maintain SpO_2 > 94% and $PaCO_2$ 35-40 mm Hg
- Promote venous drainage (elevate head of bed 30°-45°, relieve any pressure on neck)
- Hyperosmolar therapy (mannitol, hypertonic saline 3% or 23.4%)
- Endotracheal intubation
- Hyperventilation to a $PaCO_2$ of 30 mm Hg ($EtCO_2$ of 25-30 mm Hg) for impending brain herniation
  - Avoid prolonged hypocarbia
- Optimize sedation and analgesia (propofol, midazolam, dexmedetomidine, fentanyl)
- Maintain euvolemia with 0.9% normal saline
  - Avoid overhydration
- Decompressive craniotomy for hematoma
- Early insertion of ICP monitor for CSF drainage (ventricular catheter, parenchymal probe)

SECONDARY ACTIONS

- Consider central venous access for hypertonic saline administration
  - Consider administration of hypertonic saline through a large bore peripheral IV if central line unavailable
- Promote mild hypothermia
- Obtain computed tomography of the head
- Avoid corticosteroids with traumatic brain injury
- Treat underlying cause

MEDICATIONS

- 3% hypertonic saline: 150-250 mL IV infusion over 30 minutes
- 23.4% hypertonic saline: 30 mL IV bolus over 10 minutes
- Consider a 3% hypertonic saline infusion of 30 mL/h if three or more 3% hypertonic saline boluses have been administered within 6 hours
- Avoid hypertonic saline if serum sodium is above 155 mEq/L
- Mannitol 0.25-1 g/kg one time

- Vasopressor(s) to maintain MAP > 80 mm Hg (caution in patients with intracerebral hemorrhage):
  - Phenylephrine 50-100 mcg IV bolus, 0.1-0.5 mcg/kg/min infusion and/or,
  - Norepinephrine 5-10 mcg IV bolus, 0.1-0.5 mcg/kg/min infusion and/or,
  - Vasopressin 1-2 Unit IV bolus, 0.01-0.05 Units/min infusion
- Acetazolamide 150-250 mg PO twice daily for high-altitude cerebral edema

PHYSIOLOGY AND PATHOPHYSIOLOGY

Intracranial pressure (ICP) is the pressure exerted on brain tissue within the skull. The Monro-Kellie principle describes the cranial vault as a rigid box that cannot expand. Therefore, the contents within the cranial vault (brain tissue, cerebral spinal fluid [CSF], extracellular fluid, and blood) are relatively fixed, although blood and CSF can vary depending on ICP. The etiology of increased ICP can be narrowed into intracranial (primary) and extracranial (secondary) causes, increased CSF production, decreased CSF re-sorption, and increases in cerebral blood volume (see Table 20-1).

Normal ICP is ≤ 15 mm Hg, thus and intracranial hypertension occurs when ICP is > 20 mm Hg. Cerebral perfusion pressure (CPP) is the net pressure gradient that drives blood flow and subsequently oxygen delivery to brain tissue cells. It is calculated by subtracting the ICP from the mean arterial blood pressure (MAP). The calculation is CPP = MAP − ICP. Cerebral autoregulation is the brain's ability to regulate cerebral blood flow over a wide range of arterial pressures (60-140 mm Hg). Normal cerebral blood flow is 40 to 60 mL per 100 grams of brain tissue per minute.

Brain injury interrupts normal cerebral autoregulation causing cerebral blood flow to become pressure dependent. When elevated ICP causes a reduction in CPP, perfusion to brain tissue is decreased resulting in cerebral tissue hypoxia and potential infarction. Furthermore, as ICP increases, brain tissue structures are at risk of either supratentorial and or infratentorial herniation and brainstem compression. The physiologic response to decreased cerebral perfusion is (1) a systemic increase in MAP, and (2) cerebral vaso dilation. A concerning cycle of increased cerebral blood flow, additional increases in ICP and resulting decreases in CPP can result.

Table 20-1 Causes of Increased ICP

Intracranial (primary) causes	• Traumatic brain injury from blunt or penetrating trauma causing epidural or subdural hematomas, brain tissue contusions, or intracerebral hemorrhage • Stroke causing intracerebral infarct and brain tissue swelling • Brain tumor • Nontraumatic intracerebral hemorrhage (e.g., aneurysm rupture) • Idiopathic intracranial hypertension • Infections such as encephalitis or meningitis, ruptured cerebral vessel with bleeding in the brain • High-altitude cerebral edema
Extracranial (secondary) causes	• Hypoventilation leading to hypoxia and hypercarbia • Hypertension • Seizures • Hyperpyrexia • High-altitude cerebral edema
Increased CSF production	• Idiopathic increase in CSF production • Choroid plexus tumor
Decreased CSF Resorption	• Obstructive hydrocephalus • Meningeal inflammation or granulomas
Increases in cerebral blood volume	• Increased cerebral blood flow from hypercarbia or pharmacological treatments (e.g., inhalation anesthetics, vasodilators) • Venous sinus thrombosis • Elevated central venous pressures
Other causes	• Skull deformities (e.g., craniosynostosis) • Hypervitaminosis A (Vitamin A toxicity) • Tetracycline antibiotic use

Rapid identification and intervention of elevated ICP is important for improved patient outcomes. First, a thorough medical history can help to identify potential causes of increased ICP. Neurological signs and symptoms include headache, visual changes, altered level of consciousness, and pupillary changes. The use of point of care ultrasound (POCUS) targeting the optic nerve can help to identify papilledema, which is swelling around the optic nerve (> 6 mm) caused by elevated ICP. Temporizing measures can be employed to maintain and possibly decrease ICP. Definitive treatment consists of insertion of an ICP monitor (intraventricular catheters are considered the gold standard), CSF drainage, and either surgical or medical correction of the cerebral insult.

SIGNS AND SYMPTOMS

Neurologic

- Altered level of consciousness
- Coma (late finding)
- Headache
- Hemiparesis
- ICP > 15 mm Hg
- Nausea, vomiting
- Papilledema (can be visualized with POCUS)
- Seizure activity
- Visual problems: blurred vision, diplopia, dilated pupils with minimal to no reaction to light

Respiratory

- Shallow respirations
- Irregular respirations are a late sign of increased ICP

Cardiovascular

- Hypertension (later sign shows wide pulse pressure)
- Tachycardia or bradycardia
- Dysrhythmias

Other considerations

- Cushing's triad is a late sign of increased ICP: hypertension (widening pulse pressure), bradycardia, and irregular deep respirations
- Generalized weakness
- Neck rigidity

DIFFERENTIAL DIAGNOSIS

Neurologic

- Acute cardiovascular accident
- Acute nerve injury
- Hydrocephalus
- Intracranial hemorrhage
- Intracranial epidural abscess or hematoma
- Meningioma
- Migraine variants
- Subarachnoid hemorrhage or hematoma

Respiratory

• Severe hypoxia

Cardiovascular

• Heart block
• Hypertensive crisis
• Vasovagal reaction

Pharmacologic

• Acute sympathomimetic drug misuse (e.g., cocaine, methamphetamine)
• Acute alcohol or depressant drug intoxication
• Drug error (e.g., excessive phenylephrine, epinephrine, norepinephrine, or vasopressin administration)

Other considerations

• Eclampsia (associated with pregnancy)
• High altitude
• Lyme disease

Diagnostic tests

• Intracranial pressure monitoring using intraventricular catheter, intraparenchymal probe, or subarachnoid bolt
• POCUS ocular nerve assessment
• Computed tomography of the head
• Electrolyte panel, coagulation studies, hemoglobin/hematocrit

Suggested Readings

• Bonanno LS. Neuroanatomy, neurophysiology, and neuroanesthesia. In: Elisha S, Heiner JS, Nagelhout JJ, eds. *Nurse Anesthesia.* 7th ed. St. Louis: Elsevier; 2023:502-504.
• Changa AR, Czeisler BM, Lord AS. Management of elevated intracranial pressure: a review. *Curr Neurol Neurosci Rep.* 2019;19(12):99.
• Marehbian J, Muehlschlegel S, Edlow BL, Hinson HE, Hwang DY. Medical management of the severe traumatic brain injury patient. *Neurocrit Care.* 2017;27(3):430-446.
• Sookplung P, Siriussawakul A, Malakouti A, et al. Vasopressor use and effect on blood pressure after severe adult traumatic brain injury. *Neurocrit Care.* 2011;15(1):46-54.

CHAPTER 21   High/Total Spinal Anesthesia

MANAGEMENT

PRIMARY ACTIONS

- Treatment is supportive until the level of the blockade and/or the cerebral concentration of local anesthetic decreases
- Provide left uterine displacement for parturients
- If the patient is conscious, administer 100% oxygen, provide reassurance, and assess the spinal level (e.g., dermatome, ability to squeeze their hand, ability to phonate)
- If there is loss of consciousness and/or inadequate respiratory effort, provide mask ventilation with 100% oxygen
- Secure and maintain a patent airway
- Assess and maintain an appropriate blood pressure
  1. IV fluid bolus
  2. Vasopressor(s) for hypotension (see "Medications")
  3. Use phenylephrine with caution since it can exacerbate bradycardia
  4. Consider vasopressin in the presence of refractory hypotension
- Administer atropine for profound bradycardia (see "Medications")
- Perform ACLS or PALS per American Heart Association protocol

MEDICATIONS

- Vasopressor(s) to maintain MAP > 65 mm Hg:
  - Ephedrine 5-10 mg IV bolus and/or,
  - Phenylephrine 50-100 mcg IV bolus, 0.1-0.5 mcg/kg/min infusion and/or,
  - Epinephrine 10-100 mcg IV bolus, 0.1-0.5 mcg/kg/min infusion and/or,
  - Dopamine 5-20 mcg/kg/min IV infusion and/or,
  - Norepinephrine 5-10 mcg bolus, 0.1-0.5 mcg/kg/min infusion and/or,
  - Vasopressin 1-4 Unit bolus, 0.01-0.1 Units/min infusion
- For severe bradycardia
  - Atropine 0.5-1 mg IV bolus

PHYSIOLOGY AND PATHOPHYSIOLOGY

Diffusion of high concentrations of local anesthetic (LA) medications during spinal anesthesia can spread excessively cephalad (high spinal anesthesia) and eventually into the brain (total spinal anesthesia). High, or total, spinal anesthesia results in profound bradycardia, hypotension, loss of consciousness, cardiac/respiratory arrest, and death. Specific causes that can result in high, or total, spinal anesthesia include:

1. Epidural catheter migration into the subarachnoid space causes unintentional excessive concentrations of LA in the subarachnoid space
2. Excessive LA administration into the epidural space via the epidural needle or catheter
3. Excessive LA administration into the subarachnoid space during spinal anesthesia
4. Inadvertent placement of an epidural needle or catheter into the subarachnoid space—puncture causes unintentional excessive concentrations of LA in the subarachnoid space
5. Subdural injection
6. Use of a hypobaric solution for spinal anesthesia.
7. Valsalva maneuver is initiated when the patient holds their breath, bears down, and/or strains while attempting to change positions. The Valsalva maneuver causes a decreased venous return to the heart, epidural vein engorgement, increased pressure on the dura mater, and increased pressure within the subarachnoid space. This increased pressure within the subarachnoid space can lead to the cephalad spread of increased concentrations of local anesthesia into the brain.

The severity of the signs and symptoms is dependent on the level of motor, sensory, and sympathetic nerve fiber blockade. Severe hypotension can occur due to profound blockade of B preganglionic sympathetic nerve fibers. Phrenic nerve function originates at the C3-C5 nerve roots and allows for diaphragmatic contraction and breathing. The cardioaccelerator nerve fibers arise from the T1-T4 spinal nerve roots and transmit efferent impulses that maintain sympathetic nervous system input to the heart. Cephalad spread of LA that migrates above these vertebral segments can result in apnea and/or profound bradycardia/asystole, respectively.

SIGNS AND SYMPTOMS

Neurologic

- Altered level of consciousness/unconsciousness
- Anxiety
- Feeling of an inability to breathe
- Nausea/vomiting
- Seizures

Respiratory

- Aphonia
- Decreased SpO_2
- Difficulty breathing
- Dyspnea
- Respiratory depression/arrest

Cardiovascular

- Bradycardia if spinal nerve block extends at or above the T1 nerve root
- Cardiac arrest
- Dysrhythmias
- Hypotension
- Tachycardia

Other considerations

- Difficulty phonating/talking
- Dysphagia
- Unable to squeeze hands and/or move upper extremities

DIFFERENTIAL DIAGNOSIS

Neurologic

- Bezold-Jarisch reflex
- Cerebrovascular accident

Seizures respiratory

- Hypoxia
- Vasoplegic

Cardiovascular

- Aortocaval compression
- Celiac reflex
- Hypovolemia
- Myocardial ischemia/infarction
- Refractory hypotension

Pharmacologic

- Local anesthetic toxicity

Other considerations

- Hypoglycemia
- Subarachnoid injection
- Subdural injection
- Spinal cord infarction

Suggested Readings

- Asfaw G, Eshetie A. A case of total spinal anesthesia. *Int J Surg Case Rep.* 2020;76:237-239.
- Pellegrini JE, Conley RP. Regional anesthesia: spinal and epidural anesthesia. In: Elisha S, Heiner JS, Nagelhout JJ, eds. *Nurse Anesthesia.* 7th ed. St. Louis: Elsevier; 2023:1109-1140.
- Sisay A, Girma B, Negusie T, Abdi S, Horsa B, Ayele K. Inadvertent life-threatening total spinal anesthesia following caudal block in a preschool child underwent urologic surgery: a rare case report. *Int J Surg Case Rep.* 2021;88:106541. doi:10.1016/j.ijscr.2021.106541.

CHAPTER 22   Anaphylactic Shock

MANAGEMENT

PRIMARY ACTIONS

- Discontinue suspected causative agent(s)
- Maintain patent and secure airway with adequate ventilation (consider early intubation if airway edema is present)
- Monitor for the presence of rapidly developing airway edema and obstruction
- Administer 100% FiO_2
- Discontinue anesthetic medication
- Administer fluid bolus to treat hypotension
- Administer epinephrine IV or IM (see "Medications")
- Follow ACLS and PALS guidelines as indicated

SECONDARY ACTIONS

- Invasive monitoring (arterial line), as necessary
- Monitor and treat acid-base abnormalities
- Consider ICU admission

MEDICATIONS

- Epinephrine 10-100 mcg IV bolus or 300 to 500 mcg IM, can repeat every 5 to 15 minutes (or more frequently), as needed
- Antihistamine: diphenhydramine (Benadryl) 0.5-1 mg/kg IV
- H2 blocker: famotidine (Pepcid) 20 mg IV after Benadryl administration
- Bronchodilators for persistent bronchospasm:
  - Albuterol 2.5 to 5 mg by nebulization every 20 minutes for three doses, or give 4 to 8 puffs by metered dose inhaler (with spacer) every 20 minutes for 3 doses
  - Ipratropium bromide (Atrovent) 500 mcg via nebulizer every 20 minutes for 3 doses, or 4 to 8 puffs by metered dose inhaler every 20 minutes for 3 doses
  - Terbutaline 0.25 mg SC injection every 20 minutes times 3 doses
  - Magnesium sulfate 40-50 mg/kg IV, or IV infusion 2 grams over 20 minutes
- Hydrocortisone 150 to 200 mg IV or decadron 4-8 mg IV
- Sodium bicarbonate 0.5-1 mEq/kg IV for persistent hypotension or acidosis
- Vasopressor(s) to maintain MAP > 65 mm Hg:
  - Ephedrine 5-10 mg IV bolus and/or,
  - Phenylephrine 50-100 mcg IV bolus, 0.1-0.5 mcg/kg/min infusion and/or,
  - Epinephrine 10-100 mcg IV bolus, 0.1-0.5 mcg/kg/min infusion and/or,
  - Dopamine 5-20 mcg/kg/min IV infusion and/or,
  - Norepinephrine 5-10 mcg bolus, 0.1-0.5 mcg/kg/min infusion and/or,
  - Vasopressin 1-4 Unit bolus, 0.01-0.1 Units/min

PHYSIOLOGY AND PATHOPHYSIOLOGY

Anaphylaxis is a type 1, immune-mediated hypersensitivity reaction caused by the degranulation of sensitized mast cells and basophils after exposure to an antigen. Mast cells are located in the perivascular spaces of the skin, lung, and intestine, whereas basophils are located in the blood. On initial exposure to an antigen, immunoglobulin E (IgE) is produced and binds to the surface of the effector cell. With subsequent exposure, the antigen binds to the IgE antibodies, releasing physiologically active mediators that include histamine, tryptase, chemotactic factors, and platelet-activating factor. Furthermore, metabolites such as prostaglandins, kinins, leukotrienes, and cytokines are synthesized and released. When released, these active mediators and metabolites cause potentially life-threatening symptoms, most notably in the respiratory, cardiovascular, and integumentary systems. An anaphylactic reaction can occur during the first exposure to anesthetic medications from cross-reactivity among many drugs and commercial household products.

In an anaphylactoid reaction (nonimmunologic hypersensitivity reaction), IgE is not produced, but the offending agent (e.g., drug, food) causes direct degranulation of mast cells and basophils. No previous sensitization is needed to trigger anaphylactoid reactions, and the physiologic effects are clinically indistinguishable from the signs and symptoms associated with anaphylaxis. The time of onset and the degree of clinical manifestations can vary greatly, making diagnosis complicated. In addition, many symptoms may be masked by general anesthesia and surgical drapes, which conceal the cutaneous signs. Table 22-1 lists the agents that most commonly cause

Table 22-1 Allergens implicated in causing anaphylaxis

AGENT	INCIDENCE (%)
• Neuromuscular blocking agents	58.2
• Latex	16.7
• Antibiotics	15.1
• Colloids	4.0
• Hypnotics	3.4
• Opioids	1.3
• Other agents (e.g., chlorhexadine, IV contrast, protamine)	1.3
• Sugammadex	0.08

anaphylaxis. Epinephrine is the drug of choice for anaphylaxis as it inhibits the degranulation of histamine releasing cells and increases vascular resistance and cardiac contractility.

SIGNS AND SYMPTOMS

Respiratory

- Acute respiratory failure
- Altered breath sounds
- Bronchospasm
- Changes in voice quality
- Chest discomfort
- Coughing
- Cyanosis
- Decreased oxygen saturation
- Dyspnea
- Increased end-tidal carbon dioxide
- Sloped expiratory limb of end-tidal carbon dioxide waveform
- Increased peak inspiratory pressures
- Laryngeal/oral edema
- Sneezing
- Wheezing

Cardiovascular

- Cardiac arrest
- Chest discomfort
- Diaphoresis
- Dizziness
- Dysrhythmias
- Hypotension
- Tachycardia

Other considerations

- Flushing
- Itching
- Perioral edema
- Periorbital edema
- Urticaria (hives and/or rash)
- Tingling

DIFFERENTIAL DIAGNOSIS

Respiratory

- Airway obstruction
- Bronchospasm
- Hypoxia

- Laryngospasm
- Pneumothorax
- Pulmonary edema
- Pulmonary embolism
- Stridor

Cardiovascular

- Cardiac dysrhythmias
- Cardiac tamponade
- Hereditary angioedema
- Hypotension
- Myocardial ischemia/infarction
- All shock states
- Vasovagal reaction
- Venous air embolism

Gastrointestinal

- Acute gastric aspiration
- Esophageal or endobronchial intubation

Pharmacologic

- Direct histamine release (morphine sulfate, atracurium)
- Discontinuation or overdose of vasoactive drug infusion
- Local anesthetic toxicity
- Medication error causing hypotension

Other considerations

- Acute generalized urticaria and/or angioedema
- Electrolyte abnormalities
- Systemic/cutaneous mastocytosis
- Mast cell activation syndrome

Diagnostic tests

- Mast cell tryptase levels 30 minutes after the anaphylactic episode

Suggested Readings

- Kalangara J, Vanijcharoenkarn K, Lynde GC, McIntosh N, Kuruvilla M. Approach to perioperative anaphylaxis in 2020: updates in diagnosis and management. *Curr Allergy Asthma Rep.* 2021;21(1):4.
- Moss J. Allergic to anesthetics. *Anesthesiology.* 2003;99(3):521-523.
- Roche BTH. The immune system and anesthesia. In: Elisha S, Heiner JS, Nagelhout JJ, eds. *Nurse Anesthesia.* 7th ed. St. Louis: Elsevier; 2023:1049-1075.
- Volcheck GW, Hepner DL. Identification and management of perioperative anaphylaxis. *J Allergy Clin Immunol Pract.* 2019; 7(7):2134-2142.

CHAPTER 23 Cardiac Compressive Shock

MANAGEMENT

PRIMARY ACTIONS

- Maintain normal or slightly elevated heart rate
- Hemodynamic goals:
  - Maintain preload
  - Avoid increases in afterload
  - Maintain or increase contractility
  - Maintain heart rate (avoid bradycardia)
- Increase FiO_2 to keep $SpO_2 > 90\%$
- Arterial line insertion
- Place two large-bore peripheral IV lines
- Avoid increases in intrathoracic pressure (e.g., avoid PEEP, high peak inspiratory pressures)
  - Attempt to relieve cardiac compression (e.g., drain pericardial effusion) before intubation
  - The combination of positive-pressure ventilation and sedation can result in cardiovascular collapse
  - Consider awake intubation to maintain negative pressure ventilation
  - Consider low tidal volumes and higher respiratory rates for ventilation
- Perform cardiac resuscitation per American Heart Association ACLS/PALS protocol as necessary
- Curative surgical interventions:
  - Emergency percutaneous pericardiocentesis guided by echocardiography or fluoroscopy
  - Surgical treatment (e.g., pericardiotomy by median sternotomy or anterolateral thoracotomy)

SECONDARY ACTIONS

- Assess and treat primary cause
- Consider central line placement for venous pressure and fluid administration
- Consider the presence other injuries if cardiac tamponade is associated with trauma

MEDICATIONS

- Vasopressor(s) and inotropic medications to maintain MAP > 65 mm Hg are used as a bridge to pericardiocentesis:
  - Ephedrine 5-10 mg IV bolus and/or,
  - Epinephrine 10-100 mcg IV bolus, 0.1-0.5 mcg/kg/min infusion and/or,

- Dopamine 5-20 mcg/kg/min IV infusion and/or,
- Dobutamine 0.5-5 mcg/kg/min IV infusion and/or,
- Norepinephrine 5-10 mcg IV bolus, 0.1-0.5 mcg/kg/min infusion
• Consider ketamine or etomidate for IV induction agent

PHYSIOLOGY AND PATHOPHYSIOLOGY

Cardiac compressive shock is a reversible shock state that can cause significant cardiovascular compromise and result in decreased organ perfusion. It is caused by an outside force applying pressure on the cardiac muscle, leading to reduced diastolic filling. Several factors are known to cause cardiac compressive shock including cardiac tamponade (most common), tension pneumothorax, and more rare conditions such as a rupture of the diaphragm with herniation of intraabdominal contents into the chest cavity or significant intra-abdominal pressure.

Cardiac tamponade is the result of pressure on the heart that inhibits cardiac filling and left ventricular end diastolic volume. This pathology is most commonly caused by pericardial effusion, which is an accumulation of fluid within the pericardial sack surrounding the heart. Pericardial effusions can result from an imbalance of fluid production and reabsorption, or from structural abnormalities that allow excessive fluid to accumulate within the pericardial sack. The increase in pericardial pressure causes diastolic dysfunction, leading to an increase in central venous pressure and a decrease in preload and cardiac output. Surgical procedures that are associated with cardiac tamponade include: cardiac catheterization, cardiac revascularization, and pacemaker insertion.

The rate of fluid accumulation within the pericardial space determines the speed and severity of cardiac dysfunction. Normal pericardial fluid consists of 25 to 50 mL, and a rapid accumulation of only 100 to 200 mL can cause cardiac tamponade. However, with gradual accumulation of pericardial fluid, the pericardial fibers stretch to compensate for this increased volume. When a critical volume is reached, cardiac tamponade will occur. Pericardial tamponade results in cardiovascular collapse when a drop in the arterial pressure reaches a level that does not allow for coronary artery perfusion.

Cardiac tamponade may also occur as a result of a traumatic injury (e.g., blunt force/penetrating trauma to the thorax, acceleration-deceleration injuries). Bleeding within the pericardial sack can originate from a laceration of coronary arteries or from perforation of the heart. Immediate surgical intervention is necessary to avoid cardiovascular collapse.

SIGNS AND SYMPTOMS

Neurologic

- Altered mental status
- Loss of consciousness

Respiratory

- Cyanosis
- Dyspnea
- Orthopnea
- Tachypnea

Cardiovascular

- Beck triad
    1. Hypotension
    2. Jugular venous distention
    3. Muffled heart sounds
- Cardiac arrest
- Cardiac dysrhythmias
- Chest pain or pressure
- Chest radiograph shows an enlarged cardiac shadow that appears globular
- Diastolic pressure equalization in all four cardiac chambers
- Electrocardiogram changes (e.g., evidence of ischemia)
- Echocardiography reveals fluid accumulation around the heart and diastolic collapse of the right atrium and right ventricle
- Increased central venous pressure (early sign)
- Narrowed pulse pressure
- Pulseless electrical activity
- Pulses paradoxus (decrease in systolic pressure of greater than 10 mm Hg during inspiration is a very useful sign of cardiac compressive shock)
- Syncope
- Tachycardia

Musculoskeletal

- Fatigue
- Weakness

Renal

- Oliguria

DIFFERENTIAL DIAGNOSIS

Respiratory

- Pulmonary edema
- Tension pneumothorax

Cardiovascular

- Acute myocardial ischemia or infarction
- Aortic dissection
- Cardiogenic shock
- Congestive heart failure
- Increased intrathoracic pressure (e.g., PEEP)
- Superior vena cava syndrome

Musculoskeletal

- Connective tissue disorders
- Mediastinal mass

Pharmacologic

- Anaphylaxis

Other considerations

- All shock states
- Bacterial infections (e.g., tuberculosis)
- Trauma to the chest, or severe acceleration/deceleration injuries

Diagnostic tests

- Echocardiogram is the most sensitive diagnostic exam
    - Diastolic right atrial and ventricular collapse
    - Dilated inferior vena cava with minimal or no collapse during inspiration
- Electrocardiogram
- Cardiac ultrasound
- Chest radiograph and/or computed tomography scan
- Arterial blood gas

Suggested Readings

- Elisha S. Cardiovascular anatomy, physiology, pathophysiology, and anesthesia management. In: Elisha S, Heiner JS, Nagelhout JJ, eds. *Nurse Anesthesia.* 7th ed. St. Louis: Elsevier; 2023:502-504.
- Spodick DH. Acute cardiac tamponade. *N Engl J Med.* 2003; 349:684-690.
- Ristić AD, Imazio M, Adler Y, et al. Triage strategy for urgent management of cardiac tamponade: a position statement of the European Society of Cardiology Working Group on Myocardial and Pericardial Diseases. *Eur Heart J.* 2014;35(34):2279-2284.

MANAGEMENT

PRIMARY ACTIONS

- Call for help and obtain the crash cart
- Administer 100% FiO_2 if there is evidence of hypoxia
- Obtain a 12-lead electrocardiogram
- Consult a cardiologist
- Determine the primary cause

SECONDARY ACTIONS

- Arterial line placement and obtain arterial blood gas analysis
- Chest radiograph
- Obtain serial laboratory analysis (e.g., electrolytes, cardiac markers, complete blood count, lactate)
- Facilitate timely coronary revascularization, if possible
- Consult with cardiologist to determine the need for mechanical circulatory support device:
  - Intra-aortic balloon pump
  - Impella
  - Left ventricular assist device

TREATMENT BASED ON PRIMARY CAUSE
MYOCARDIAL ISCHEMIA/INFARCTION

- Aspirin 325 mg PO (NG or OG tube)
- Nitroglycerine IV or sublingual if no hypotension
- Beta blockade (e.g., esmolol) if tachycardia present without hypotension
- Consider fibrinolytic therapy
- If STEMI, provide PCI within 12 hours of symptom onset

INCREASED AFTERLOAD

- Vasodilate with clevidipine, hydralazine, or nitrates (See "Medications")

DYSRHYTHMIA

- Determine rhythm and treat based on ACLS guidelines

VOLUME OVERLOAD

- IV fluid restriction
- Furosemide (Lasix) 40 mg IV

EXCESSIVE MYOCARDIAL DEPRESSION

- Decrease/turn off inhalational agent, turn off propofol infusion
- Consider epinephrine, dopamine, or dobutamine infusion (See "Medications")

MEDICATIONS
- Vasodilators:
  - Hydralazine 1-20 mg IV bolus and/or,
  - Nitroglycerine 5-100 mcg/min IV infusion or,
  - Nitroprusside 0.2-5 mcg/kg/min IV infusion (maximum infusion rate 10 mcg/kg/min) or,
  - Clevidipine start 1-2 mg/h IV infusion and titrate additional 1-2 mg/h until BP goal is reached (maximum 32 mg/h)
- Vasopressor(s) to maintain MAP > 65 mm Hg:

FIRST-LINE AGENTS:
  - Norepinephrine 5-10 mcg IV bolus, 0.01-0.5 mcg/kg/min infusion and/or,
  - Phenylephrine 50-100 mcg IV bolus, 0.1-0.5 mcg/kg/min infusion and/or,
  - Dobutamine 2-20 mcg/kg/min IV infusion (do not exceed 40 mcg/kg/min)

SECOND-LINE AGENTS:
  - Epinephrine 10-100 mcg IV bolus, 0.1-0.5 mcg/kg/min infusion and/or,
  - Dopamine 2-20 mcg/kg/min IV infusion and/or,
  - Vasopressin 1-2 Unit IV bolus, 0.01-0.05 Units/min infusion

PHYSIOLOGY AND PATHOPHYSIOLOGY

The pathophysiologic manifestations associated with cardiogenic shock include a reduction in cardiac contractility and stroke volume, increased intracardiac pressures, impaired coronary perfusion, cardiac ischemia that may or may not show ST changes, systemic hypotension, and inadequate end-organ perfusion. End-organ hypoperfusion triggers the release of catecholamines and vasopressin in an effort augment myocardial contractility and provide peripheral vasoconstriction. However, these neurohormonal changes only work in the short term because increases in afterload cause the heart to work harder, increasing oxygen demand and severely straining already injured myocardial tissue. If untreated, a cycle of continued myocardial ischemia, reduced cardiac output, and end-organ hypoperfusion occurs, eventually resulting in multisystem failure.

The most common cause of cardiogenic shock is acute myocardial infarction (MI) from occlusion of one or more coronary arteries. Depending on the site of ischemia and myocardial dysfunction, either right or left ventricular failure can result, causing systemic hypotension, pulmonary congestion, systemic venous congestion, and ultimately tissue hypoperfusion.

Mechanical complications of an acute MI are less common but can also lead to cardiogenic shock. An inferoposterior infarct can cause rupture of chordae tendineae or papillary muscle connected to the mitral leaflet resulting in mitral regurgitation. Anterior or inferior infarction can cause a mechanical rupture of the interventricular septum. Finally, rupture of the left ventricular free wall can lead to cardiac tamponade and significant hemorrhage. Each of these potential mechanical complications can progress to cardiogenic shock.

Noncardiac causes can contribute to cardiogenic shock. Hypovolemic shock caused by a decreased amount of circulating blood volume can ultimately contribute to a reduction in coronary perfusion leading to cardiogenic shock. Obstructive shock, such as cardiac tamponade, limits the ability of the heart to contract effectively causing a reduction in CO and stroke volume. Distributive shock (e.g., anaphylaxis) limits the amount of venous return, decreasing CO and stroke volume. In addition, patients with septic shock are at risk for developing cardiogenic shock because of the severe reduction in venous return and coronary perfusion. Because of the systemic inflammatory response, there is an upregulation of inducible nitric oxide synthase, which ultimately results in pathological amounts of nitric oxide (NO). The large amount of circulating NO causes systemic vasodilation, a decrease in venous return, inhibition of cardiac inotropy, impaired coronary perfusion, and reduced CO.

SIGNS AND SYMPTOMS

Neurologic

- Altered or decreased level or consciousness
- Anxiety

Respiratory

- Cyanosis
- Dyspnea/tachypnea
- Hypercarbia
- Hypoxia
- New-onset rales

Cardiovascular

- Compensated cardiogenic shock: hypertension/tachycardia
- Uncompensated cardiogenic shock: hypotension/bradycardia
- Arrhythmia
- Chest pain

- Decreased peripheral and central pulses
- Delayed capillary refill
- Diaphoresis
- ECG changes: ST segment elevation or depression
- Elevated troponin levels
- Jugular venous distention
- Pallor
- Wall motion abnormalities on TEE

Urologic

- Decreased urine output (oliguria)

Other considerations

- Metabolic acidosis
- Lactate > 2 .0 mmol/L

DIFFERENTIAL DIAGNOSIS

Neurologic

- Increased ICP with signs of impending herniation (e.g., dysrhythmias, blood pressure abnormalities)

Respiratory

- Tension pneumothorax

Cardiovascular

- Pulmonary embolism

Endocrine

- Acute adrenal insufficiency
- Carcinoid syndrome

Pharmacologic

- Medication error (e.g., beta-blockade overdose)

Other considerations

- Any other shock state (e.g., sepsis, anaphylaxis, hypovolemia)
- High intraabdominal pressure (e.g., pneumoperitoneum with rapid and high insufflation pressure)

Diagnostic tests

- Arterial blood gas
- Cardiac markers: troponin
- Chest radiograph
- Coronary angiography and ventriculography

- Electrocardiogram
- Laboratory analysis: electrolytes, complete blood count, lactate
- Transesophageal echocardiography
- Transthoracic echocardiography

Suggested Readings

- Elisha S. Cardiovascular anatomy, physiology, pathophysiology, and anesthesia management. In: Elisha S, Heiner JS, Nagelhout JJ, eds. *Nurse Anesthesia*. 7th ed. St. Louis: Elsevier; 2023:502-504.
- Hochman JS, Sleeper LA, Webb JG, et al. Early revascularization in acute myocardial infarction complicated by cardiogenic shock. SHOCK Investigators. Should we emergently revascularize occluded coronaries for cardiogenic shock. *N Engl J Med*. 1999;341(9):625-634.
- Shah AH, Puri R, Kalra A. Management of cardiogenic shock complicating acute myocardial infarction: a review. *Clin Cardiol*. 2019;42(4):484-493.
- Vahdatpour C, Collins D, Goldberg S. Cardiogenic shock. *J Am Heart Assoc*. 2019;8(8):e011991.

CHAPTER 25 Hypovolemic Shock (Acute Hemorrhage)

MANAGEMENT

PRIMARY ACTIONS

- Call for help and obtain the crash cart
- Administer 100% FiO_2 and ensure patent airway
- Establish multiple large bore IV acess (consider central line or Intraossious line as indicated)
- Treat underlying pathological state
- Ensure surgical management/intervention
  1. Direct (manual) pressure to the wound or surgical site
  2. Use of topical hemostatic agents
  3. Surgical ligation or clamping of blood vessels
- Initiate goal-directed fluid therapy with crystalloid, colloid, factor concentrates, and blood product component therapy (administration based on clinical and laboratory assessment)
- Avoid lethal triad: acidosis, hypothermia, and coagulopathy

SECONDARY ACTIONS

- Supportive measures as necessary
  1. Airway management and mechanical ventilation
  2. Invasive monitoring (e.g., arterial pressure, central venous pressure)
  3. Monitor acid-base, fluid, and electrolyte balance
  4. Consider vasopressor(s) administration for severe hypotension (see "Medications")
- Activate goal-directed massive transfusion protocol.
  - For example, 4 units packed red blood cells + 4 units fresh frozen plasma + 1 pooled platelet unit (e.g., equal to 4-6 individual units).
    - Consider adjunctive therapeutic agents (e.g., antifibrinolytics)
- Type and cross
- Baseline arterial blood gas analysis
- Baseline hemoglobin, hematocrit, platelet, and electrolyte values (particulary potassium and calcium)
- Obtain fibrinogen level
- Autologous blood cell salvage and autotransfusion (confirm surgical site is not contaminated or cancerous)
- Consider lower extremetiy elevation or head down position (e.g., Trendelenburg position)

MEDICATIONS

- Antifibrinolytics
  - Aminocaproic acid 4-5 gram IV loading dose given over 1 hour, then 1 gram/h infusion for 8 hours and/or,

- Tranexamic acid (TXA) 10-30 mg/kg IV given over 10-30 minutes
  • TXA should be considered in patients with a history of blunt or penetrating trauma who are at risk of massive hemorrhage and should be administered within 3 hours of trauma injury.
• Calcium chloride: 1 gm IV over 10 minutes (if hypocalcemic)
• Recombinant Factor VIIa 70 to 90 mcg/kg/dose IV, every 2-3 hours until hemostasis is achieved
  - Avoid in patients with coagulopathy, hypothermia, or acidosis
• Vasopressor(s) to maintain MAP > 65 mm Hg:
  - Ephedrine 5-10 mg IV bolus and/or,
  - Phenylephrine 50-100 mcg IV bolus, 0.1-0.5 mcg/kg/min infusion and/or,
  - Epinephrine 10-100 mcg IV bolus, 0.1-0.5 mcg/kg/min infusion and/or,
  - Dopamine 5-20 mcg/kg/min IV infusion and/or,
  - Norepinephrine 5-10 mcg IV bolus, 0.1-0.5 mcg/kg/min infusion and/or,
  - Vasopressin 1-4 Unit IV bolus, 0.01-0.1 Units/min infusion

PHYSIOLOGY/PATHOPHYSIOLOGY

Hypovolemia is a decreased circulating blood volume, resulting in anemia. The World Health Organization has defined anemia as a hemoglobin concentration of less than 13 g/dL for adult males and less than 12 g/dL for adult, nonpregnant females. Causes of perioperative anemia include: (1) decreased erythrocyte production, (2) increased erythrocyte loss, (3) increased erythrocyte destruction, and/or (4) decreased serum hemoglobin concentration. Undiagnosed anemia is the most common hematological problem during preoperative patient management. Preoperative anemia can indicate an underlying pathological state or condition that may affect surgical outcomes. Before major elective surgery, it is prudent to identify and treat anemia in order to optimize hemoglobin levels (e.g., iron supplementation, erythropoietic-stimulating agents).

Hypovolemic shock occurs when severe intravascular volume depletion decreases blood flow to vital organs. It is classified into two types: nonhemorrhagic and hemorrhagic. Nonhemorrhagic hypovolemic shock results from significant fluid loss such as severe vomiting, diarrhea, urinary loss (e.g., diabetes insipidus), or sweating. Hemorrhagic hypovolemic shock occurs because of blood loss from traumatic or surgical rupture of the vasculature. Hemorrhagic hypovolemic shock is the most common type of shock in the trauma patient population.

Decreased circulating blood volume, resulting in low perioperative hemoglobin, reduces the oxygen-carrying capacity of the blood. It increases the risk of morbidity and mortality in patients with cardiac, respiratory, and neurovascular disease. Medical management of acute anemia (e.g., acute hemorrhage) should attempt to: (1) maintain hemodynamic stability, (2) maximize blood oxygen-carrying capacity, and (3) maximize oxygen delivery to peripheral and central tissues.

Allogeneic blood transfusions are not without risk and can cause (1) viral transmission, (2) bacterial contamination, (3) transfusion-related acute lung injury, (4) transfusion-related cardiac overload, and (5) acute transfusion reactions. Recommendations for allogeneic blood transfusion include:

- Transfusion is not warranted when the hemoglobin concentration is greater than 10 g/dL, unless there is evidence of inadequate perfusion, oxygenation, and/or significant comorbidities
- Transfusion is indicated when the hemoglobin concentration is less than 6 g/dL
- When the hemoglobin concentrations are between 6 and 10 g/dL, the decision to transfuse is determined by:
  1. Evidence of organ ischemia (e.g., hypotension, dysrhythmias)
  2. Actual or potential bleeding
  3. Presence of risk factors that cause inadequate oxygenation (e.g., decreased cardiopulmonary reserve)

SIGNS AND SYMPTOMS

Neurologic
- Altered level or loss of consciousness
- Confusion
- Fatigue
- Restlessness

Respiratory
- Congestive heart failure
- Dyspnea and tachypnea
- Hemoptysis
- Hypercarbia
- Hypoxia
- Pulmonary edema

Cardiovascular
- Angina pectoris
- Arterial waveform amplitude variation with respiration

- Decreased peripheral and/or central pulses with decreased capillary refill time
- Dysrhythmias
- Low and/or narrow pulse pressure
- Low central venous pressure
- Low left ventricular end-diastolic pressure
- Myocardial infarction or ischemia
- Orthostatic hypotension
- Palpitations
- Pulse oximetry plethysmographic waveform amplitude variation with respiration
- Systemic hypotension
- Tachycardia

Renal

- Hematuria
- Oliguria

Hematologic

- Hemoglobin concentration of less than 13 g/dL for adult males and less than 12 g/dL for adult, nonpregnant females

Gastrointestinal

- Hematemesis
- Hematochezia
- Hepatosplenomegaly
- Melena

Musculoskeletal

- Bone pain

Other considerations

- Integumentary
  1. Pallor of skin and mucous membranes
  2. Petechiae
  3. Purpura
- Physical examination
  1. Lymphadenopathy
  2. Metabolic acidosis (e.g., lactic acidosis)
  3. Menstrual blood loss

DIFFERENTIAL DIAGNOSIS

Respiratory

- Cystic and cavitary pulmonary disease (e.g., tuberculosis)
- Goodpasture syndrome

- Lung cancer
- Pulmonary embolus

Cardiovascular

- Hypotension
- Retroperitoneal bleeding (e.g., discoloration of the flank region)
- Rupture of major blood vessels from trauma
- Ruptured aneurysm (e.g., aortic or cerebral)

Renal

- Renal disease

Endocrine

- Acute adrenal crises
- Hypoadrenalism
- Hypopituitarism
- Hypothyroidism

Hematologic

- Aplastic anemia (e.g., Fanconi or Diamond-Blackfan syndromes)
- Hemolytic anemia potential causes:
  1. Autoantibodies transfusion reaction
  2. Autoimmune mediated
  3. Disseminated intravascular coagulation
  4. Erythrocyte cell membrane disorder (e.g., hereditary spherocytosis or elliptocytosis)
  5. Erythrocyte enzymopathy (e.g., glucose-6-phosphate dehydrogenase deficiency)
  6. Erythrocyte pyruvate kinase deficiency
  7. Hemoglobin Hammersmith
  8. Hemolytic uremic syndrome
  9. Infection mediated
  10. Microangiopathic hemolytic anemia
  11. Paroxysmal nocturnal hemoglobinuria
  12. Prosthetic heart valve
  13. Sickle cell disease
  14. Thrombotic thrombocytopenic purpura
- Iron deficiency anemia
- Megaloblastic anemia
  1. Folate deficiency
  2. Vitamin B12 deficiency
- Myeloproliferative disorder
- Thalassemia

Gastrointestinal

- Colon cancer
- Colonic diverticula or diverticulitis
- Esophageal varices
- Esophagogastric mucosal laceration (e.g., Mallory-Weiss Syndrome)
- Gastric and duodenal ulcers
- Gastritis
- Liver disease

Pharmacologic

- Acute alcohol intoxication or withdrawal
- Anticonvulsant therapy
- Antithrombotic medication (e.g., antiplatelet, anticoagulant, or fibrinolytic)
- Chemotherapy reaction
- Exogenous allergens (e.g., penicillin allergy)
- Methemoglobinemia
- Sulfhemoglobinemia

Other considerations

- Anemia of chronic disease
  1. Hypersplenism
  2. Metastatic cancer
- Mechanical origin
  1. Disconnected intra-arterial device (e.g., arterial line, aortic cannula, and intra-aortic balloon catheter)
- Obstetrical or gynecological origin
  1. Abruptio placenta
  2. Obstetric hemorrhage resulting from uterine atony
  3. Placenta accreta, increta, or percreta
  4. Placenta previa
  5. Ruptured ectopic pregnancy
  6. Ruptured ovarian cyst
  7. Uterine rupture
- Traumatic injury
  1. Blunt trauma to the thorax or abdomen
  2. Extensive burn injury
  3. Laceration(s) to major vessels
  4. Penetrating injury (e.g., gunshot wounds, stab wounds, and projectiles)

Diagnostic tests

- Arterial blood gas
- Complete blood count

- D-dimer
- Fibrinogen
- Functional hemodynamic monitoring (e.g., stroke volume variation, pulse pressure variation, Pleth variability index)
- Prothrombin time, activated partial thromboplastin time, activated clotting time
- Serum electrolyte test(s): sodium, potassium, calcium, magnesium
- Thromboelastogram
- Type and screen/crossmatch
- Ultrasound assessment of inferior vena cava collapsibility

Suggested Readings

- American Society of Anesthesiologists Task Force on Perioperative Blood Management. Practice guidelines for perioperative blood management: an updated report by the American Society of Anesthesiologists Task Force on Perioperative Blood Management. *Anesthesiology*. 2015;122(2):241-275. doi:10.1097/ALN.0000000000000463.
- Brazzel C. Thromboelastography-guided transfusion therapy in the trauma patient. *AANA J*. 2013;81(2):127-132.
- Collins S, MacIntyre C, Hewer I. Thromboelastography: clinical application, interpretation, and transfusion management. *AANA J*. 2016;84(2):129-134.
- Howie WO. Trauma anesthesia. In: Elisha S, Heiner JS, Nagelhout JJ, eds. *Nurse Anesthesia*. 7th ed. St. Louis: Elsevier; 2023:930-949.

CHAPTER 26 Neurogenic Shock

MANAGEMENT

PRIMARY ACTIONS

- Administer 100% oxygen and ensure patent airway
- Airway management as needed with rapid sequence induction (maintain in-line manual axial stabilization and remove C-collar during airway management)
  - Use lung protective ventilation 6-8 mL/kg and Pplat < 30 cm H_2O
  - Maintain oxygen saturation > 90%
- Aggressively manage hypotension:
  - Obtain a minimum two large-bore peripheral IV lines
  - IV fluid bolus 10-20 mL/kg isotonic crystalloid
  - Vasopressors/atropine as needed (See "Medications")
- Maintain cervical spine precautions
- Forced air warming
- External cardiac pacing
- Arterial line placement
- Rule out other causes of shock (e.g., hypovolemic, cardiogenic, cardiac compressive)

SECONDARY ACTIONS

- Initiate ACLS or PALS as needed
- Serial laboratory values: arterial blood gas, electrolytes, lactate, complete blood count
- Neurology consultation
  - Perform American Spinal Injury Association (ASIA) impairment assessment to evaluate level of function below spinal cord injury (see Table 26-1)
- If placing a central venous catheter, consider using the subclavian vein if a cervical collar is present
- Foley catheter
- Deep vein thrombosis prophylaxis
- Pressure sore protection
- Provide warming measures

MEDICATIONS

- Vasopressor(s) to maintain MAP between 85 and 90 mm Hg (to improve spinal cord perfusion):
  First-line agents:
  - Norepinephrine 5-10 mcg IV bolus, 0.1-0.5 mcg/kg/min infusion and/or,
  - Phenylephrine 50-100 mcg IV bolus, 0.1-0.5 mcg/kg/min infusion (AVOID IF BRADYCARDIA IS PRESENT)
  - Epinephrine 10-100 mcg IV bolus, 0.1-0.5 mcg/kg/min infusion and/or,

Second-line agents:
- Dopamine 2-20 mcg/kg/min IV infusion and/or,
- Vasopressin 1-2 Unit IV bolus, 0.01-0.05 Units/min infusion
• Atropine 0.4-1 mg IV bolus or glycopyrrolate 0.4 mg (especially before tracheal suctioning)

Table 26-1 American Spinal Injury Association (ASIA) standard neurological classification of spinal cord injury impairment score

CATEGORY	DESCRIPTION
A - Complete	No motor or sensory function is preserved in the sacral segments S4-S5
B - Incomplete	Sensory but not motor function is preserved below the neurological level and includes the sacral segments S4-S5
C - Incomplete	Motor function is preserved below the neurological level, and more than half of key muscles below the neurological level have a muscle grade of < 3 on the AISA motor score (against gravity without additional resistance)
D - Incomplete	Motor function is preserved below the neurological level, and at least half of the key muscles below the neurological level have a muscle grade ≥ 3 on the ASIA motor score (antigravity)
E - Normal	Motor and sensory function are normal

PHYSIOLOGY AND PATHOPHYSIOLOGY

Neurogenic shock primarily occurs from damage to the spinal cord, resulting from a combination of primary and secondary injuries causing a loss of sympathetic tone and unopposed parasympathetic (vagal) response. This sympathectomy can result in significantly unstable blood pressure caused by vasodilation, blood pooling within the peripheral circulation, and decreased venous return. A high spinal cord injury (above T6) can also cause profound brady-cardia from a loss of cardioaccelerator activation and a subsequent inability to increase cardiac output. There is some discussion that neurogenic shock can present with substantial hypotension and *without* bradycardia if the level of injury is below T6. Preganglionic sympathetic neurons originate in the intermediolateral cell column of the spinal cord between T1 and L2. Therefore, an injury *below* the level of the cardioaccelerator fibers (T1-T4) may cause widespread peripheral vasodilation but a preservation of the patient's innate ability to compensate with an increase in heart rate. Temperature dysregulation follows because sympathetic pathways are interrupted between the hypothalamus and peripheral blood vessels resulting in profound vasodilation.

Trauma is a leading cause of spinal cord injury. Primary spinal cord injury results from direct damage to the spinal cord. Traumatic vertebral fractures or dislocations cause compression or transection of spinal cord neural tissue such as neural axons, oligodendrocytes, white or gray matter, spinal tracts, and/or sensory and motor roots. Neurogenic shock occurs when damaged spinal cord neural tissue disrupts sympathetic tone, such as the intermediolateral nucleus of the lateral gray column and/or preganglionic visceral motor fibers that exit the spinal cord in the anterior nerve root. These tracts originate at the first thoracic vertebrae and extend to either the second or third lumbar vertebra.

Secondary spinal cord injury can occur several hours or days after the initial injury. These injuries are associated with hypoperfusion to spinal cord neural tissue from edema, arterial thrombosis, vasospasm, and/or vascular destruction at the site of injury. Both controlled and uncontrolled programmed cell death (apoptosis) can occur at the spinal cord cellular level from altered perfusion, electrolyte shifts (primarily calcium and potassium), mitochondrial injury, and reperfusion injury. In addition, hemorrhage disrupts the blood–spinal cord barrier and exposes the spinal cord to inflammatory cells (macrophages, neutrophils, and lymphocytes), cytokines, vasoactive peptides and vascular hematomas, which can remain within the spinal cord exacerbating tissue swelling and spinal cord compression.

Other nontraumatic causes of neurogenic shock include autonomic nervous system toxins, Guillain-Barré syndrome, high spinal anesthesia, or transverse myelitis.

SIGNS AND SYMPTOMS

Neurologic

- Altered level of consciousness or loss of consciousness
- Anxiety
- Dizziness
- Loss of sensation in upper and/or lower extremities
- Nausea and/or vomiting
- Spinal tenderness

Respiratory

- Apnea from diaphragmatic denervation (level C3-C5)
- Cyanosis
- Dyspnea/tachypnea
- Hypercarbia
- Hypoxia
- Slow respiratory rate

Cardiovascular

- Autonomic dysreflexia
- Bradyarrhythmia (distinctive sign)
- Chest pain
- Decreased peripheral and/or central pulses
- Dysrhythmias (heart block)
- Heart block/asystole from cardio-accelerator denervation (level T1-T4)
- Hypotension
- Orthostatic hypotension
- Warm flushed extremities
- Widening pulse pressure

Other considerations

- Hypothermia
- Loss of bowel or bladder tone
- Metabolic acidosis

DIFFERENTIAL DIAGNOSIS

Neurologic

- Increased intracranial pressure
- Spinal shock
- Transverse myelitis

Respiratory

- Hypoxia (severe)

Cardiovascular

- Heart block
- Myocardial infarction
- Venous air or gas embolism

Pharmacologic

- Acute intoxication
- Medication error

Other considerations

- All shock states (hypovolemic, obstructive, cardiogenic, septic, anaphylactic)
- Electrolyte abnormalities (hypocalcemia, hyponatremia, hyperkalemia)
- Guillain-Barré syndrome
- High spinal anesthesia

Diagnostic tests

- Computed tomography of the spine
- Computed tomography angiography to evaluate vertebral artery integrity
- Clinical evaluation of spine
- Hemodynamic monitoring
- Magnetic resonance imaging for evaluation of soft tissue structures (vertebral ligaments, intervertebral discs, spinal cord, nerve roots)

Suggested Readings

- Ahuja CS, Wilson JR, Nori S, et al. Traumatic spinal cord injury. *Nat Rev Dis Primers*. 2017;3:17018.
- Alizadeh A, Dyck SM, Karimi-Abdolrezaee S. Traumatic spinal cord injury: an overview of pathophysiology, models and acute injury mechanisms. *Front Neurol*. 2019;10:282.
- Dave S, Cho JJ. Neurogenic shock. [Updated 2022 Feb 10]. In: *StatPearls* [Internet]. Treasure Island, FL: StatPearls Publishing; 2022. Available at: https://www.ncbi.nlm.nih.gov/books/NBK459361/.
- Howie W. Trauma anesthesia. In: Elisha S, Heiner JS, Nagelhout JJ, eds. *Nurse Anesthesia*. 7th ed. St. Louis: Elsevier; 2023:930-949.
- Guly HR, Bouamra O, Lecky FE, Trauma Audit and Research Network. The incidence of neurogenic shock in patients with isolated spinal cord injury in the emergency department. *Resuscitation*. 2008;76(1):57-62.
- Standl T, Annecke T, Cascorbi I, Heller AR, Sabashnikov A, Teske W. The nomenclature, definition and distinction of types of shock. *Dtsch Arztebl Int*. 2018;115(45):757-768.

CHAPTER 27   Septic Shock

MANAGEMENT

PRIMARY ACTIONS

- Administer 100% oxygen and ensure patent airway
- Administer broad-spectrum antibiotic within 1 hour of diagnosis (see "Medications")
- Obtain large-bore IV access
- Maintain mean arterial pressure (MAP) > 65 mm Hg by:
  - 30 mL/kg IV initial bolus of isotonic crystalloid (maximum = 80 mL/kg)
  - Norepinephrine infusion (see "Medications")
  - Add vasopressin infusion after volume replacement and if norepinephrine alone does not achieve target MAP (see "Medications")
  - Consider albumin if large crystalloid volumes are being infused
  - Avoid IV starches (e.g., hetastarch)
- If hypotension continues, despite vasopressor therapy, administer:
  - Hydrocortisone 200 mg IV bolus
- Intubation and mechanical ventilation
  - Tidal volume 6-8 mL/kg
  - Plateau pressures < 30 cm H_2O
  - PEEP 5 cm H_2O minimum
- Maintain blood glucose < 180 mg/dL
- Remove infected/necrotic tissue that may be the source of septic shock

SECONDARY ACTIONS

- Arterial line placement
- Consider central line placement (maintain CVP at 8-12 mm Hg)
- Type and screen
- Serial laboratory values: arterial blood gas, electrolytes, lactate, complete blood count, coagulation panel
- Obtain bacterial cultures: wound, blood, urine, stool, cerebrospinal fluid
- Consultation with intensivist and admission to intensive care unit within 6 hours of diagnosis
- Assess for hypovolemia (goal-directed fluid therapy)
- Venous thromboembolism prophylaxis with low molecular weight heparin
- Remove and replace potential sources of infection (e.g., central line, Foley catheter)
- Initiate ACLS or PALS as needed

MEDICATIONS

- Broad-spectrum IV antibiotics
  - Piperacillin-tazobactam (Zosyn) 3.375 g IV every 6 hours

- Ceftriaxone (Rocephin) 1-2 g IV every day
- Vancomycin 15-20 mg/kg IV infusion every 12 hours at a rate of 10 mg/min for at least 1 hour
- Vasopressor(s) to maintain MAP > 65 mm Hg:
  - Primary agents:
    - Norepinephrine 5-10 mcg IV bolus, 0.1-0.5 mcg/kg/min infusion and/or,
    - For progressive shock – Epinephrine 10-100 mcg IV bolus, 0.1-0.5 mcg/kg/min infusion and/or,
  - Secondary agents:
    - Vasopressin 1-2 Unit IV bolus, 0.01-0.05 Units/min infusion and/or,
    - Dopamine 5-20 mcg/kg/min IV infusion

PHYSIOLOGY AND PATHOPHYSIOLOGY

Sepsis, as defined by the surviving sepsis campaign, results in life-threatening organ dysfunction caused by a "dysregulated" response to infection. Its clinical progression follows a spectrum that begins with systemic inflammatory response syndrome (SIRS) and can result in multiorgan dysfunction syndrome (MODS) and death. How an individual progresses is influenced by their overall health and rapid multidisciplinary management. The most common cause of sepsis syndromes are gram-negative bacterial infections followed by gram-positive infections. At the vascular level, endothelial dysfunction causes:

1. An alteration in vascular tone, resulting in vasodilation and hypotension affecting oxygen delivery to cells.
2. Impaired distribution of intravascular volume with vascular permeability that diminishes microcirculation, because of capillary leak resulting in reduced oxygen distribution.
3. Dysfunctional mitochondria causing altered oxygen processing eventually leading to anaerobic metabolism and lactic acidosis.

The body's response to an offending pathogen causes activation of both pro-inflammatory and anti-inflammatory immune system activity. Immune cells such as monocytes, macrophages, and neutrophils interact with pathogen recognition receptors on the vascular endothelium, which stimulates the release of cytokines, kinins, proteases, reactive oxygen species, and nitric oxide. Activation of the coagulation and complement cascades occurs with microvascular endothelial injury. Histamine, serotonin, super-radicals, and lysosomal enzymes are released as a result of bacterial endotoxins. The consequences of a systemic wide infection and hyperactive immune response are significant reductions in vascular compliance, impaired microcirculation, reduced oxygenation, lactic acidosis, and end-organ dysfunction.

Activation of the inflammatory, complement, and coagulation cascades results in the symptoms associated with sepsis and septic shock. The body's ability to regulate pro-inflammatory responses that eliminate microorganisms, while also balancing anti-inflammatory signals responsible for overall control of the inflammatory cascade, influences an individual's morbidity and mortality from sepsis.

Septic shock is the most severe complication resulting from sepsis. It is commonly caused by hypovolemia, impaired cardiovascular function, mitochondrial dysfunction, and coagulopathy (both pro- and anti-coagulation types). Mortality from septic shock is higher depending on the degree of organ injury (e.g., respiratory, cardiovascular, neurologic, hepatic, and/or renal failure).

SIGNS AND SYMPTOMS

Early (compensated) signs and symptoms:

- ***Neurologic***
  - Fever (> 38° C)
  - Anxiety
  - Altered level of consciouness
- ***Respiratory***
  - Tachypnea (> 20 breaths/min)
- ***Cardiovascular***
  - Flash capillary refill (< 1 second)
  - Normal to elevated BP
  - Tachycardia with bounding pulses (greater than 90 beats/min)
  - Warm and flushed

Progressive (uncompensated) signs and symptoms:

- ***Neurologic***
  - Altered level of consciousness or loss of consciousness
- ***Respiratory***
  - Possible acute respiratory distress syndrome
  - Cyanosis
  - Dyspnea/tachypnea
  - Hypercarbia and hypoxia
- ***Cardiovascular***
  - Decreased capillary refill with cool extremities
  - Decreased peripheral pulses
  - Dysrhythmias
  - Hypotension
  - Possible myocarditis
  - Tachycardia

- *Renal*
  - Acute kidney injury
  - Decreased glomerular filtration rate
  - Elevated serum blood urea nitrogen and creatinine
  - Oliguria and/or anuria
- *Other Considerations*
  - Adrenal gland insufficiency
  - Coagulopathy (e.g., disseminated intravascular coagulation)
  - Gastrointestinal ileus
  - Increased temperature
  - Leukocytosis (white blood cell [WBC] count greater than 12,000/cu mm) or leukopenia (WBC less than 4000/cu mm)
  - Metabolic acidosis
  - Serum lactate (elevated in early and progressive shock)

DIFFERENTIAL DIAGNOSIS

Neurologic

- Encephalitis
- Increased intracranial pressure
- Meningitis

Respiratory

- Acute respiratory distress syndrome
- Pulmonary embolism

Cardiovascular

- Heart failure

Endocrine

- Acute adrenal insufficiency
- Carcinoid syndrome
- Diabetic ketoacidosis
- Pancreatitis

Pharmacologic

- Medication error
- Medication or toxin overdose/withdrawal

Other considerations

- All other shock states (anaphylactic, neurogenic, cardiogenic, cardiac compressive, hypovolemic)
- Bowel obstruction
- Disseminated intravascular coagulation
- Toxic shock syndrome

Diagnostic tests

- Arterial blood gas
- Computed tomography of the chest and abdomen
- Cultures of wound, blood, urine, and cerebrospinal fluid
- Echocardiogram
- Elevated mixed venous oxygen saturation (> 70%)
- Laboratory analysis:
    - CBC (thrombocytopenia - platelets < 100,000/mL; leukocytosis -WBC > 12×10^9/L; or leukopenia - WBC < 4×10^9/L)
    - Coagulation abnormalities (INR > 1.5 or PTT > 60 s)
    - Cortisol level low (< 150 µg/L)
    - Electrolyte abnormalities
    - Elevated serum lactate (> 2 mmol/L)
    - Hyper- or hypoglycemia
    - Liver function abnormalities
- PaO_2: FiO_2 ratio < 300
- Radiograph of chest
- Specialized laboratory studies: C-reactive protein or procalcitonin more than 2 standard deviations above normal
- Ultrasound as indicated

Suggested Readings

- Elisha S. Cardiovascular anatomy, physiology, pathophysiology, and anesthesia management. In: Elisha S, Heiner JS, Nagelhout JJ, eds. *Nurse Anesthesia*. 7th ed. St. Louis: Elsevier; 2023:502-504.
- Evans L, Rhodes A, Alhazzani W, et al. Surviving sepsis campaign: international guidelines for management of sepsis and septic shock 2021. *Intensive Care Med.* 2021;47(11):1181-1247.
- Gyawali B, Ramakrishna K, Dhamoon AS. Sepsis: The evolution in definition, pathophysiology, and management. *SAGE Open Med.* 2019;7:2050312119835043.
- Hotchkiss RS, Moldawer LL, Opal SM, Reinhart K, Turnbull IR, Vincent JL. Sepsis and septic shock. *Nat Rev Dis Primers*. 2016;2:16045.
- Polat G, Ugan RA, Cadirci E, Halici Z. Sepsis and septic shock: current treatment strategies and new approaches. *Eurasian J Med.* 2017;49(1):53-58. doi:10.5152/eurasianjmed.2017.17062.
- Standl T, Annecke T, Cascorbi I, Heller AR, Sabashnikov A, Teske W. The nomenclature, definition and distinction of types of shock. *Dtsch Arztebl Int.* 2018;115(45):757-768.

CHAPTER 28 Acute Renal Dysfunction

MANAGEMENT

PRIMARY ACTIONS

- Determine and treat the underlying cause (e.g., all shock states, hypovolemia, nephrotoxic drugs, endogenous toxins)
- Maintain adequate blood pressure (MAP $\geq$ 70 mm Hg) and end-organ perfusion:
  1. Correct hypovolemia with balanced crystalloid volume resuscitation (administer lactated ringers or Plasma-Lyte in 250-1000 mL boluses)
  2. Maintain systemic vascular resistance with vasopressor(s) (see "Medications")
  3. Consider type and crossmatch for blood product administration if warranted
  4. If bleeding time is increased, consider the administration of platelets, FFP, cryoprecipitate, or desmopressin before surgery
- Avoid nephrotoxic medications:
  1. Nonsteroidal anti-inflammatory medications
  2. Angiotensin-converting enzyme inhibitor and angiotensin receptor blockers
  3. Aminoglycoside antibiotics
  4. Radiographic contrast dye

SECONDARY ACTIONS

- Consider invasive monitoring (e.g., arterial/central line)
- Review laboratory results and manage appropriately (e.g., complete blood count, coagulation, electrolytes, renal function, glucose and HbA1c, urine creatinine clearance, and urine protein)
- Place a urinary catheter to monitor urine output
- Avoid diuretics unless needed to treat volume overload
- Consultation with a nephrologist and a cardiologist
- Renal replacement therapy as indicated:
  1. Dialysis
  2. Peritoneal dialysis
  3. Hemofiltration
  4. Kidney transplantation

MEDICATIONS

- Vasopressor(s) and inotropic agents to maintain MAP $>$ 70 mm Hg:
  - Ephedrine 5-10 mg IV bolus and/or,

- Dopamine 1-5 mcg/kg/min IV infusion and/or,
- Norepinephrine 5-10 mcg IV bolus, 0.1-0.5 mcg/kg/min infusion and/or,
- Vasopressin 1-4 Units IV bolus, 0.01-0.1 Units/min infusion

PHYSIOLOGY AND PATHOPHYSIOLOGY

Acute renal dysfunction, also known as acute kidney injury or acute renal failure, occurs when there is a sudden decline in glomerular filtration. This can occur over a period of hours or days, and is usually reversible when the cause is identified and treated. Those at highest risk for acute renal dysfunction are elderly patients with concurrent comorbidities (e.g., hypertension, diabetes) and any baseline renal insufficiency.

Acute renal dysfunction is divided into three pathophysiologic categories: (1) prerenal, (2) intrarenal, and (3) postrenal (see Table 28-1). These pathophysiologic categories represent causes of renal dysfunction that encompass hypoperfusion of the kidney, damage or toxic exposure to the renal parenchyma, or acute obstruction of the urinary tract.

The abrupt deterioration in renal function alters the kidney's ability to excrete nitrogenous waste products as well as maintain adequate fluid and electrolyte homeostasis. As a result, there is a severe decrease in the glomerular filtration of the blood, an elevation in serum blood urea nitrogen and creatinine (> 0.3 mg/dL), an accumulation of other metabolic waste products that are normally excreted by the kidney, and either a decrease or cessation of urine output.

SIGNS AND SYMPTOMS

Neurologic

- Confusion
- Headache
- Lethargy
- Seizure

Respiratory

- Dyspnea
- Tachypnea
- Pulmonary edema

Cardiovascular

- Fatigue
- Dysrhythmias from electrolyte (e.g., hyperkalemia) and/or acid-base abnormalities

Table 28-1 Pathophysiology and etiology associated with acute renal dysfunction

	PATHOPHYSIOLOGY	ETIOLOGY
Prerenal causes	Decreased renal blood flow	1. Acute hemorrhage (e.g., "trauma, surgery, postpartum delivery, gastrointestinal system) 2. Intravascular volume depletion (e.g., diarrhea, vomiting, burns, osmotic diuresis, diabetes insipidus) 3. Aortic cross clamping/dissecting aorta 4. Arteriosclerosis 5. Congestive heart failure 6. Decreased cardiac output 7. Hypotension 8. Hypovolemia 9. Large third space loss (e.g., ascites, postburn) 10. Renal artery stenosis or disease 11. All shock states
Intrarenal causes	Direct damage to renal parenchyma	1. Glomerular injuries (e.g., glomerulonephritis, other renal inflammatory conditions, hematologic disorders) 2. Acute tubular necrosis (e.g., caused by ischemia, nephrotoxic medications, radiographic contrast dye, endogenous toxins such as rhabdomyolysis or myoglobinuria) 3. Interstitial nephritis 4. Preeclampsia 5. Renal vascular disease
Postrenal causes	Decrease in forward flow of urine leading to hydronephrosis and an interruption in normal kidney function	1. Retroperitoneal or bladder tumors 2. Catheter obstruction or kink 3. Pelvic or intraabdominal tumors 4. Prostatic hypertrophy 5. Renal calculi (kidney stones)

- Chest pain
- Hypovolemia
- Hypervolemia
- Hypertension
- Orthostatic hypotension
- Tachycardia

Hematologic

- Anemia
- Coagulopathy

Renal

- Acute decrease in glomerular filtration rate
- Increases in serum creatinine concentrations
- Decreased urine output (< 0.3-0.5 mL/kg/h for 6-12 hours)

Hepatic

- Decreased hepatic function and altered metabolism of drugs
- Hepatic vascular congestion

Gastrointestinal

- Nausea and/or vomiting
- Weight loss

Integumentary

- Lower extremity swelling

DIFFERENTIAL DIAGNOSIS

Neurologic

- Acute cerebrovascular accident
- Postoperative cognitive dysfunction

Respiratory

- Pulmonary edema

Cardiovascular

- Congestive heart failure
- Dysrhythmias
- Myocardial infarction
- Hypotension
- Hypovolemia

Renal

- Acute renal dysfunction conditions (see Table 28-1)
  - Prerenal (reduced blood flow to the kidney)

  - Intrarenal (direct kidney tissue injury)
  - Postrenal (urinary flow obstruction)
- Nephrotic syndrome
- Obstructed foley catheter
- Prior renal dysfunction or existing renal problems

Hepatic

- Cirrhosis

Hematologic

- Anemia
- Blood transfusion reaction
- Coagulopathy

Musculoskeletal

- Rhabdomyolysis

Other considerations

- Hyperkalemia
- Major operative procedures with large amounts of blood loss or decreased renal perfusion (e.g., cardiopulmonary bypass, abdominal aortic aneurysm repair)
- Multiorgan dysfunction syndrome
- Sepsis
- Trendelenburg position can cause anuria because of pooling of urine in the bladder

Diagnostic tests

- Increased serum creatinine $\geq$ 0.3 mg/dL
- Acute decrease in glomerular filtration rate > 25%
- Electrolyte abnormalities (e.g., hyperkalemia, hypocalcemia)

Suggested Readings

- Morse CY. Renal anatomy, physiology, pathophysiology, and anesthesia management. In: Elisha S, Heiner JS, Nagelhout JJ, eds. *Nurse Anesthesia*. 7th ed. St. Louis, MO: Saunders Elsevier; 2023:742-769.
- Gumbert SD, Kork F, Jackson ML, et al. Perioperative acute kidney injury. *Anesthesiology*. 2020;132:180-204.
- Goren O, Matot I. Perioperative acute kidney injury. *Br J Anaesth*. 2015;115:ii3-ii14.

CHAPTER 29 Electrolyte Abnormalities

MANAGEMENT

PRIMARY ACTIONS:

- Treat neurologic, cardiac, respiratory, and neuromuscular manifestations
- Treat underlying pathological causes
- Consider electrolyte-specific replacement for total body deficits
- See Table 29-1 for management of particular electrolyte abnormalities
- Follow current ACLS/PALS guidelines

SECONDARY ACTIONS:

- Supportive measures, as necessary (see "Medications")
  1. Airway management and mechanical ventilation
  2. Invasive monitoring (e.g., arterial, central venous catheter)
  3. Monitor acid-base, fluid, and electrolyte balance and obtain appropriate laboratory analysis as indicated

MEDICATIONS:

- Antidysrhythmics, follow current ACLS/PALS guidelines
- Vasopressor(s) to maintain MAP > 65 mm Hg:
  - Ephedrine 5-10 mg IV bolus and/or,
  - Phenylephrine 50-100 mcg IV bolus, 0.1-0.5 mcg/kg/min infusion and/or,
  - Epinephrine 10-100 mcg IV bolus, 0.1-0.5 mcg/kg/min infusion and/or,
  - Dopamine 5-20 mcg/kg/min IV infusion and/or,
  - Norepinephrine 5-10 mcg IV bolus, 0.1-0.5 mcg/kg/min infusion and/or,
  - Vasopressin 1-4 Unit IV bolus, 0.01-0.1 Units/min infusion

PHYSIOLOGY/PATHOPHYSIOLOGY

Appropriate intracellular and extracellular electrolyte concentration gradients (e.g., bution within the body: (1) fluid stat sodium, potassium, calcium, magnesium) are essential for maintaining physiologic homeostasis. Electrolyte imbalances alter cellular electrophysiology (e.g., resting membrane potential, threshold potential, action potential, and neurotransmission). Perioperative alterations in electrolyte content and distribution can produce multiorgan system dysfunction. The primary treatment of electrolyte imbalances identifies and treats the underlying pathological state.

Table 29-1 Electrolyte imbalances: symptoms, differential diagnosis, and treatment

ELECTROLYTE	SIGNS & SYMPTOMS	DIFFERENTIAL DIAGNOSIS	MANAGEMENT
Sodium (Hyponatremia)	• Serum concentration < 135 mEq/L • Altered level of consciousness • Cardiac conduction abnormalities • Cerebral edema • Increased intracranial pressure • Respiratory arrest • Seizures	• Addison disease • Brain stem herniation • Corticosteroid depletion • Excess absorption of irrigation solutions (e.g., transurethral resection of the prostate syndrome) • Gastrointestinal loss • Heart, liver, and renal failure • Hypoadrenalism • Hypothyroidism • Overhydration and/or excess water ingestion • Syndrome of inappropriate antidiuretic hormone secretion • Thiazide diuretics	• Treat pathological cause • Water restriction to < 800 mL/d • Loop-diuretics (e.g., furosemide) • Hypertonic saline (3% or 5%), 1-2 mL/kg/r not to exceed 100 mL/h

Continued

Table 29-1 Electrolyte imbalances: symptoms, differential diagnosis, and treatment—cont'd

ELECTROLYTE	SIGNS & SYMPTOMS	DIFFERENTIAL DIAGNOSIS	MANAGEMENT
Sodium (Hypernatremia)	• Serum concentration > 145 mEq/L • Ascites • Decreased urine output • Hypotension and tachycardia • Increased blood urea nitrogen and creatinine • Increased urine-specific gravity • Pleural effusion	• Corticosteroid excess • Cushing disease • Dehydration and/or decreased water ingestion • Diabetes insipidus • Hyperventilation • Osmotic diuretics • Renal failure (e.g., impaired sodium excretion)	• Treat pathological cause • Electrolyte-free water (5% glucose in water), maximum rate of correction 0.5 mEq/L/h • Potassium-sparing diuretics (e.g., spironolactone)

Table 29-1 Electrolyte imbalances: symptoms, differential diagnosis, and treatment—cont'd

ELECTROLYTE	SIGNS & SYMPTOMS	DIFFERENTIAL DIAGNOSIS	MANAGEMENT
Postassim (Hypokalemia)	• Serum concentration < 3.5 mEq/L • Cardiac dysrhythmias (e.g., U wave, flattened or inverted T wave) • Digoxin toxicity • Orthostatic hypotension • Skeletal muscle weakness	• Antibiotics (e.g., penicillin analogs and aminoglycosides) • Cushing disease • Diuretics (e.g., thiazide and loop diuretics) • Gastrointestinal loss • Hyperaldosteronism • Hyperglycemia • Insulin overdose • Mineralocorticoid and glucocorticoids drugs • Respiratory/metabolic alkalosis • β-adrenergic agonists	• Treat pathological cause • Potassium replacement for true deficit, maximum rate of replacement 20 mEq/h (0.2 mEq/kg/h)

Continued

Table 29-1 Electrolyte imbalances: symptoms, differential diagnosis, and treatment—cont'd

ELECTROLYTE	SIGNS & SYMPTOMS	DIFFERENTIAL DIAGNOSIS	MANAGEMENT
Potassium (Hyperkalemia)	• Serum concentration > 5.5 mEq/L • Cardiac dysrhythmias (e.g., peaked T waves, prolonged PR interval, absent P wave, widened QRS, and ventricular arrhythmias) • Skeletal muscle weakness	• Angiotensin-converting enzyme inhibitors • Acute and chronic renal failure • Addison disease • Diuretics (e.g., spironolactone and triamterene) • Hypoaldosteronism • Nonsteroidal anti-inflammatory drugs • Respiratory or metabolic acidosis • Succinylcholine administration following: burns, spinal cord injury, crush injury, and prolonged immobilization • β-adrenergic antagonists	• Treat pathological cause • Calcium 10% chloride (10 mL over 10 min) or calcium gluconate • Glucose and insulin IV (5-10 units per 25-50 g of glucose) • Sodium bicarbonate (50-150 mEq over 5-10 min) • Beta2 agonists • Hyperventilation • Hemodialysis

Table 29-1 Electrolyte imbalances: symptoms, differential diagnosis, and treatment—cont'd

ELECTROLYTE	SIGNS & SYMPTOMS	DIFFERENTIAL DIAGNOSIS	MANAGEMENT
Calcium (Hypocalcemia)	• Serum concentration < 4.5 mEq/L • Cardiac dysrhythmias (e.g., shortened PR interval and prolonged QT interval) • Chvostek and/or Trousseau signs • Circumoral paresthesia • Hypotension • Laryngospasm • Seizures	• Acute pancreatitis • Decreased plasma albumin • Decreased serum magnesium • Hypertonic phosphate enemas • Hypoparathyroidism • Increased serum fatty acid • Renal failure • Respiratory alkalosis • Transfusion of blood products containing citrate • Vitamin D deficiency	• Treat pathological cause • Calcium replacement (e.g., 10% calcium chloride 10 mL over 10 minutes for emergency replacement; 10% calcium gluconate 10 mL over 10 min for mild/moderate symptoms) • Thiazide diuretics

Continued

Table 29-1 Electrolyte imbalances: symptoms, differential diagnosis, and treatment—cont'd

ELECTROLYTE	SIGNS & SYMPTOMS	DIFFERENTIAL DIAGNOSIS	MANAGEMENT
Calcium (Hypercalcemia)	• Serum concentration > 5.5 mEq/L • Cardiac dysrhythmias (e.g., prolonged PR interval, shortened QT interval, and ST-segment) • Digitalis toxicity • Hypertension	• Hyperparathyroidism • Immobilization • Neoplastic bone metastases • Sarcoidosis • Vitamin D toxicity	• Treat pathological cause • Hydration with normal saline • Loop diuretics (e.g., furosemide) • Bisphosphonates • Hemodialysis • Mithramycin
Magnesium (Hypomagnesemia)	• Serum concentration <1.5 mEq/L • Altered response to muscle relaxants • Cardiac dysrhythmias (e.g., torsades de pointes) • Digitalis toxicity • Hyperreflexia • Increased deep tendon reflexes • Seizures • Skeletal muscle spasms	• Chronic alcoholism • Gastrointestinal loss • Hyperalimentation therapy without magnesium • Malabsorption syndromes	• Treat pathological cause • Magnesium replacement

Table 29-1 Electrolyte imbalances: symptoms, differential diagnosis, and treatment—cont'd

ELECTROLYTE	SIGNS & SYMPTOMS	DIFFERENTIAL DIAGNOSIS	MANAGEMENT
Magnesium (Hypermagnesemia)	• Serum concentration >2.5 mEq/L • Cardiac and respiratory arrest • Coma • Depressed deep tendon reflexes • Hyporeflexia • Sedation • Skeletal muscle weakness	• Chronic renal failure • Iatrogenic (e.g., administration for pregnancy-induced hypertension and excessive use of antacids or laxatives)	• Treat pathological cause • Calcium administration • Fluid administration • Diuretics • Hemodialysis

Numerous factors influence electrolyte content and distribution within the body: (1) fluid status (e.g., total body water content and distribution); (2) acid-base status; and (3) endocrine function (e.g., hypothalamus, pituitary gland, thyroid gland, parathyroid glands, adrenal cortex, kidney). Electrolyte imbalances are often a reflection of at least one of these factors. The severity of an electrolyte imbalance is dependent on (1) etiology, (2) onset and duration (e.g., acute or chronic presentation), (3) absolute electrolyte imbalance, and (4) effects on organ function (e.g., neurologic, cardiac, respiratory, neuromuscular).

SIGNS AND SYMPTOMS

Neurologic

• Altered deep tendon reflexes
• Altered level of consciousness
• Delayed emergence from anesthesia
• Paresthesias
• Seizures

Respiratory

• Laryngospasm
• Respiratory pattern alterations (e.g., tachypnea, bradypnea)

Cardiovascular

- Altered myocardial contractility
- Cardiac conduction abnormalities
- Dysrhythmias
- Hypertension
- Hypotension
- Myocardial infarction or ischemia

Musculoskeletal

- Altered muscle contraction

Differential diagnosis

- See Table 29-1 for symptoms, differential diagnosis, and management of specific electrolyte imbalances

Diagnostic tests

- 12-lead electrocardiogram
- Arterial blood gas
- Functional hemodynamic monitoring (e.g., stroke volume variation, pulse pressure variation, Pleth variability index)
- Serum electrolyte test(s): sodium, potassium, calcium, and magnesium

Suggested Readings

- Cornelius B, Ferrell E, Kilgore P, et al. Incidence of hypocalcemia and role of calcium replacement in major trauma patients requiring operative intervention. *AANA J*. 2020;88(5):383-389.
- Khan ZH, Movafegh A, Ali HKA. Dysrhythmias under general anesthesia and their management. *Arch Anesth Crit Care*. 2019;5(3):104-106.
- McLain N, Parks S, Collins MJ. Perioperative goal-directed fluid therapy: a prime component of enhanced recovery after surgery. *AANA J*. 2021;89(4):351-357.

SECTION 7 Endocrine Emergencies

CHAPTER 30 Acute Adrenal Crisis

MANAGEMENT

PRIMARY ACTIONS

- Endotracheal intubation and controlled ventilation for respiratory arrest
- Intravascular volume expansion with lactated Ringer's or normal saline
- Administer D50W bolus for hypoglycemia
- Hydrocortisone (see "Medications")
- Treat hypotension (see "Medications")

SECONDARY ACTIONS

- Invasive monitoring (arterial line), as necessary
- Monitor laboratory values (e.g., electrolytes and glucose)
- Identify and treat the underlying cause (e.g., sepsis)
- Perform cardiac resuscitation per American Heart Association ACLS/PALS protocol as necessary

MEDICATIONS

- Hydrocortisone 100 mg IV bolus, followed by 50 mg every 6 hours for 24 hours, total: 200 mg/24 hours
- Vasopressor(s) to maintain MAP > 65 mm Hg:
  - Ephedrine 5-10 mg IV bolus and/or,
  - Phenylephrine 50-100 mcg IV bolus, 0.1-0.5 mcg/kg/min infusion and/or,
  - Epinephrine 10-100 mcg IV bolus, 0.1-0.5 mcg/kg/min infusion and/or,
  - Dopamine 5-20 mcg/kg/min IV infusion and/or,
  - Norepinephrine 5-10 mcg bolus, 0.1-0.5 mcg/kg/min infusion and/or,
  - Vasopressin 1-4 Unit bolus, 0.01-0.1 Units/min infusion

PHYSIOLOGY AND PATHOPHYSIOLOGY

The adrenal glands are located immediately superior to the kidneys. Hormones that are secreted by the adrenal cortex include (1) mineralocorticoids (primarily aldosterone), (2) glucocorticoids (primarily cortisol), and (3) androgens. Glucocorticoids exert a powerful physiologic effect on every body system. Cortisol is responsible for many physiologic reactions including: maintenance of blood sugar, fluid and electrolyte, and maintenance of normal vascular tone.

Secretion of cortisol from the adrenal cortex is dependent on the functional integrity of the hypothalamic-pituitary-adrenal axis. Primary adrenal insufficiency (Addison disease) is due to adrenocortical dysfunction. Acute adrenal insufficiency (AAI) can be caused by damage (e.g., trauma) or pathology (e.g., malignancy) to the hypothalamus, anterior pituitary, or adrenal cortex. Patients receiving exogenous steroids perioperatively may develop AAI during episodes of physiologic stress resulting from adrenal cortical atrophy. Patients taking supraphysiologic doses of exogenous steroids (e.g., prednisone > 20 mg/d or its equivalent for ≥ 3 weeks within 12 months before surgery) are considered to be at risk for developing acute adrenal crisis during the perioperative period.

A single induction dose of etomidate can cause adrenal insufficiency for up to 24 to 48 hours after its administration. The mechanism associated with etomidate induced AAI can occur from the inhibition of 11-β-hydroxylase, which is an enzyme necessary to produce cortisol. Additionally, sepsis and emergency procedures associated with a high incidence of infection can lead to acute adrenal crisis. Acute adrenal crisis is a rare but life-threatening event that must be diagnosed and treated expeditiously.

SIGNS AND SYMPTOMS

Respiratory

- Respiratory distress/arrest

Cardiovascular

- Cardiac arrest
- Dysrhythmia
- Severe hypotension minimally/unresponsive to vasopressor medications
- Tachycardia

Other considerations

- Abdominal pain
- Dizziness
- Electrolytes/glucose
  1. Hyperkalemia
  2. Hyponatremia
  3. Hypoglycemia
  4. Metabolic acidosis
- Fatigue
- Headache
- Intravascular volume depletion

- Nausea/vomiting
- Profound weakness
- Skin hyperpigmentation
- Weight loss

DIFFERENTIAL DIAGNOSIS

Cardiovascular

- All shock states
- Dysrhythmia
- Hypotension
- Hypovolemia
- Myocardial ischemia/infarction
- Vasoplegic syndrome

Endocrine

- Adrenal insufficiency

Pharmacologic

- Abrupt termination of steroid therapy
- Preoperative antihypertensive medications

Other considerations

- Medication error causing hypotension

Diagnostic tests

- Plasma adrenocorticotropic hormone stimulation test
- Serum cortisol
- Electrolyte panel

Suggested Readings

- Karlet MC. The endocrine system and anesthesia. In: Elisha S, Heiner JS, Nagelhout JJ, eds. *Nurse Anesthesia*. 7th ed. St. Louis: Elsevier; 2023:851-894.
- Liu M. Perioperative steroid management. *Anesthesiology*. 2017;127(1):166-172.
- Martin-Grace J, Dineen R, Sherlock M, Thompson CJ. Adrenal insufficiency: physiology, clinical presentation and diagnostic challenges. *Clin Chim Acta*. 2020;505:78-91.
- Możański M, Tomaszewski D, Rybicki Z, Bejm J, Bałkota M. Etomidate, but not thiopental, decreases serum cortisol concentration in morbidly obese patients. A randomized controlled trial. *Anaesthesiol Intensive Ther*. 2016;48(1):7-12.

CHAPTER 31 Diabetic Ketoacidosis

MANAGEMENT

PRIMARY ACTIONS

- Administer supplemental oxygen
- Airway management as needed
- Fluid management
  1. If hyponatremic, replace fluids using 0.9% sodium chloride at 15-20 mL/kg IV infusion in the first hour, then maintenance at 500-1000 mL/hour (maximum of < 50 mL/kg in the first 4 hours)
  2. If hypernatremic or normal serum osmolality (< 320 mOsm/kg), use 0.45% sodium chloride at 250-500 mL/hr
- Insulin administration (serum potassium ≥ 3.3 mEq/L)
  1. The goal is to decrease serum glucose by 50-100 mg/dL/h
  2. To prevent cerebral edema, do not allow the serum glucose to decrease to < 200 mg/dL
  3. See "Medications"
- Electrolytes
  1. Monitor for hyperkalemia, hypokalemia, hyponatremia, hypocalcemia, hypomagnesemia, and hypophosphatemia
  2. Monitor acid-base status and administer sodium bicarbonate for an arterial pH ≤ 7

SECONDARY ACTIONS

- Obtain 12-lead electrocardiogram
- Monitor blood glucose every 30 minutes
- Monitor electrolytes every hour
- Perform ACLS or PALS per American Heart Association protocol

MEDICATIONS

- Regular insulin 0.1-0.15 units/kg (10-20 units) IV bolus followed by, 0.1 units/kg/h infusion (5-10 units/h)

PHYSIOLOGY AND PATHOPHYSIOLOGY

Diabetic ketoacidosis (DKA) occurs when insulin deficiency causes a pathologic biochemical triad of hyperglycemia, ketonemia, and acidemia. Physiologic stress stimulates the release of hormones that increase blood glucose (e.g., cortisol, glucagon, catecholamines). Patients with diabetes have a decreased ability to secrete adequate amounts of insulin, which normally facilitates the transcellular movement and regulation of blood glucose. Consequently, during episodes of physiological stress, the lack of insulin causes lipolysis, ketogenesis, and metabolic acidosis. Furthermore, increased blood glucose and protein catabolism cause glycosuria, electrolyte depletion, and cellular dehydration. DKA is most common among people with Type 1 diabetes. However, approximately 20% of patients who present with DKA are those with undiagnosed and/or uncontrolled Type 2 diabetes. Other reasons include inadequate exogenous insulin dosing or omission, infection, and acute coronary or vascular events. Causes of DKA in patients with or without diabetes include Cushing syndrome, hyperthyroidism, pregnancy, pancreatitis, and medications (e.g., certain diuretics and corticosteroids). With prompt identification and treatment, the mortality associated with DKA in the United States is < 1%.

SIGNS AND SYMPTOMS

Respiratory

- Fruity odor on breath
- Kussmaul respirations

Cardiovascular

- Diaphoresis
- Dysrhythmias
- Orthostatic hypotension
- Tachycardia

Other considerations

- Altered level of consciousness/coma
- Electrolyte abnormalities
- Elevated blood glucose (300-800 mg/dL)
- Elevated hematocrit
- Headaches
- Hyperkalemia initially, hypokalemia after insulin therapy
- Hypochloremia
- Hyponatremia
- Ketonemia
- Metabolic acidosis (pH < 7.3 and an anion gap >15-20 mEq/L)
- Nausea
- Polydipsia
- Polyphagia
- Polyuria early, oliguria late
- Seizures
- Serum bicarbonate (≤ 18 mmol/L)

- Serum osmolality (> 300 mOsm/L)
- Weight loss

DIFFERENTIAL DIAGNOSIS

Neurologic

- Intracranial lesions
- Neuroleptic malignant syndrome

Respiratory

- Hypercarbia
- Hypoxia

Cardiovascular

- Cardiac dysrhythmias
- Cardiogenic shock
- Congestive heart failure
- Myocardial infarction

Renal

- Acute renal dysfunction

Endocrine

- Acute adrenal crises
- Hypoglycemia

Pharmacologic

- Diazoxide
- Glucocorticoids (e.g., prednisone, dexamethasone)
- Phenytoin
- Sodium-glucose Cotransporter-2 (SGLT2) Inhibitors (e.g., cana-gliflozin, empagliflozin)
- Sympathomimetics
- Thiazide diuretics

Other considerations

- Alcohol misuse and ketoacidosis
- Drug overdose (e.g., acetaminophen, aspirin, metformin)
- Fasting, starvation ketosis
- Poisoning (e.g., methanol, ethylene glycol, propylene glycol)
- Shock states

Diagnostic tests

- Arterial blood gas
- Electrolyte panel
- Glucose, blood

- Ketone level
- Serum bicarbonate
- Serum osmolality

Suggested Readings

- Dingle HE, Slovis C. Diabetic hyperglycemic emergencies: a systematic approach. *Emerg Med Pract.* 2020;22(2):1-20.
- Evans K. Diabetic ketoacidosis: update on management. *Clin Med (Lond).* 2019;19(5):396-398.
- Karlet M. The endocrine system and anesthesia. In: Elisha S, Heiner JS, Nagelhout JJ, eds. *Nurse Anesthesia.* 7th ed. St. Louis: Elsevier; 2023:851-894.
- Long B, Willis GC, Lentz S, Koyfman A, Gottlieb M. Evaluation and management of the critically ill adult with diabetic ketoacidosis. *J Emerg Med.* 2020;59(3):371-383.
- Pitocco D, Di Leo M, Tartaglione L, et al. An approach to diabetic ketoacidosis in an emergency setting. *Rev Recent Clin Trials.* 2020;15(4):278-288.

MANAGEMENT

PRIMARY ACTIONS

- Increase the anesthetic depth
- Notify the surgeon if there is sustained extreme tachycardia and/or hypertension
- Consider ending the case for uncontrolled extreme hypertension associated with undiagnosed pheochromocytoma
- See "Medications"

SECONDARY ACTIONS

- Use phenylephrine and/or vasopressin if hypotension exists after tumor resection
- Perform ACLS or PALS per American Heart Association protocol

MEDICATIONS

- Treat hypertensive crisis
  - Nicardipine 0.2-0.5 mg IV bolus, 2.5-15 mg/h infusion and/or,
  - Nitroprusside 0.2-0.5 mcg/kg/min IV infusion and/or,
  - Magnesium sulfate 1-4 g/h IV infusion and/or,
  - Clevidipine 1-20 mg/h IV infusion
- Prevent hypertensive crisis
  - First line prevention: Alpha-adrenergic blockade (goal based on age and comorbidities): phenoxybenzamine PO titrated from 10-100 mg/day over 7-14 days, *followed by*
  - Second line prevention: Beta-adrenergic blockade (goal heart rate 60 to 80 beats per minute): metoprolol PO titrated to a maximum dose of 120 mg, or metoprolol PO titrated to a maximum dose of 200 mg

PHYSIOLOGY AND PATHOPHYSIOLOGY

Pheochromocytomas are tumors that arise from the adrenal medulla. They are composed of chromaffin cells that can produce, store, and secrete catecholamines. Pheochromocytomas from the adrenal gland account for 90% of catecholamine-secreting tumors. In contrast, extra-adrenal pheochromocytomas, or catecholamine-secreting paragangliomas, can form along the paravertebral sympathetic chain or the abdominal cavity.

Pheochromocytomas most frequently affect a unilateral adrenal gland, and most are benign. Familial (or hereditary) pheochromocytomas occur in bilateral adrenal glands in 50% of cases and are frequently non-cancerous. This disease affects males and females equally and most frequently manifests between the ages of 30 and 50. There is an association between pheochromocytoma and multiple-endocrine neoplasia type II A and B, neurofibromatosis, tuberous sclerosis, Sturge-Weber syndrome, and von Hippel-Lindau disease.

Sympathetic nervous system stimulation in patients with pheochromocytoma causes a massive release of catecholamines, predominantly norepinephrine, which stimulates alpha-adrenergic receptors. Signs and symptoms associated with a pheochromocytoma include headache, diaphoresis, tachycardia, arrhythmias with palpitations, anxiety, pallor, hypertension, and hyperglycemia. Polycythemia occurs because of intravascular volume depletion resulting from extreme peripheral vasoconstriction. Cerebral hemorrhage, myocardial infarction, cardiomyopathy, congestive heart failure, and renal insufficiency can occur. Events that are associated with causing tumor activation include hypotension, hypothermia, defecation, physiologic stress, medication, intubation, and surgery.

Before surgery and anesthesia, preoperative identification and treatment are essential to avoid extreme hypertension. Alpha-adrenergic receptor blockade (phenoxybenzamine) is initially prescribed 2 weeks before surgery. Once achieved, beta-adrenergic receptor blockade is initiated to mitigate the tachycardia resulting from peripheral vascular dilation. Anesthetic

Table 32-1 Anesthetic medications to avoid in patients with pheochromocytoma

MEDICATION	EFFECT
Atracurium	Histamine release
Atropine	Sympathomimetic (tachycardia)
Desflurane	Sympathomimetic
Droperidol	Antidopaminergic-neuroleptic malignant syndrome
Ephedrine	Sympathomimetic
Ketamine	Sympathomimetic
Metoclopramide	Antidopaminergic-neuroleptic malignant syndrome
Morphine	Histamine release
Naloxone	Sympathetic nervous system predominance
Pancuronium	Sympathomimetic
Phenothiazines	Antidopaminergic-neuroleptic malignant syndrome
Succinylcholine	Fasciculations causing catecholamine release

and adjunct medications that should be avoided in a patient with a pheochromocytoma are listed in Table 32-1.

SIGNS AND SYMPTOMS

Respiratory

- Rales caused by congestive heart failure
- Shortness of breath

Cardiovascular

- Chest pain
- Diaphoresis
- Dilated cardiomyopathy
- Dysrhythmias
- Hypertension/hypertensive crises
- Orthostatic hypotension
- Tachycardia

Other considerations

- Abdominal pain
- Altered mental status
- Anxiety
- Elevated blood glucose
- Elevated hematocrit
- Headaches
- Hyperthermia
- Nausea
- Pallor
- Renal insufficiency
- Seizures

DIFFERENTIAL DIAGNOSIS

Neurologic

- Increased intracranial pressure
- Neuroleptic malignant syndrome
- Stroke

Respiratory

- Endobronchial intubation/endotracheal tube stimulating carina
- Hypercarbia
- Hypoxia

Cardiovascular

- Cardiac dysrhythmias
- Congestive heart failure

- Hypertensive crises
- Myocardial infarction
- Untreated essential hypertension

Renal

- Acute renal dysfunction

Endocrine

- Carcinoid syndrome
- Hypermetabolic syndromes (e.g., thyrotoxicosis, thyroid storm, neuroleptic malignant syndrome)

Pharmacologic

- Central anticholinergic syndrome (e.g., atropine overdose)
- Malignant hyperthermia
- Monoamine oxidase inhibitors
- Opioid and/or alcohol withdrawal
- Psychotropic medications that can cause neuroleptic malignant syndrome (e.g., haloperidol, chlorpromazine, metoclopramide, lithium)
- Sympathomimetics
  1. Drug misuse (e.g., cocaine, methamphetamine)
  2. Therapeutic medications (e.g., epinephrine)

Other considerations

- Hyperthermia
- Inadequate depth of anesthesia during surgical stimulation
- Mast cell disease
- Preeclampsia/eclampsia
- Serotonin syndrome

Diagnostic tests

- Plasma fractionated metanephrines
- 24-hour urine fractionated metanephrines and catecholamines
- Iodine-131-meta-iodobenzylguanidine scan (MIBG scan)

Suggested Readings

- Castinetti F, De Freminville JB, Guerin C, Cornu E, Sarlon G, Amar L. Controversies about the systematic preoperative pharmacological treatment before pheochromocytoma or paraganglioma surgery. *Eur J Endocrinol.* 2022;186(5):D17-D24.
- Cerqueira A, Seco T, Costa A, Tavares M, Cotter J. Pheochromocytoma and paraganglioma: a review of diagnosis, management and treatment of rare causes of hypertension. *Cureus.* 2020;12(5):e7969.

• Karlet M. The endocrine system and anesthesia. In: Elisha S, Heiner JS, Nagelhout JJ, eds. *Nurse Anesthesia*. 7th ed. St. Louis: Elsevier; 2023:851-894.
• Nölting S, Bechmann N, Taieb D, Beuschlein F, Fassnacht M, Kroiss. Personalized management of pheochromocytoma and paraganglioma. *Endocr Rev*. 2022;43(2):199-239.

CHAPTER 33 Thyroid Crisis/Storm

MANAGEMENT

PRIMARY ACTIONS

- Increase anesthetic depth
- Notify the surgeon if there is severe, sustained hypertension
- See "Medications"

SECONDARY ACTIONS

- Use phenylephrine and/or vasopressin if hypotension exists
- Hemodialysis
- Plasmapheresis
- Cholestyramine 4 g PO four times daily
- Perform ACLS or PALS per American Heart Association protocol

MEDICATIONS

- Propylthiouracil 500 mg PO or nasogastric loading dose, followed by 250 mg every 4 hours
- Sodium iodide 500 mg IV every 12 hours
- Propranolol 0.5-2 mg IV (1 mg per minute) may repeat every 2-5 minutes to a total dose of 5 mg
- Dexamethasone 4 mg IV or hydrocortisone 100 mg IV every 8 hours

PHYSIOLOGY AND PATHOPHYSIOLOGY

Early detection and prevention of thyrotoxic crisis (e.g., thyroid storm) are essential to improving patient outcomes. Resuscitative measures should be instituted as soon as possible to prevent circulatory collapse and organ system failure. During thyrotoxic crisis, the patient becomes hypermetabolic because of a precipitous increase in circulating thyroid hormone. In most cases, the diagnosis of thyroid storm is based on clinical findings alone. Because the onset of thyrotoxic crisis is abrupt, rapid treatment precludes diagnosis with laboratory tests or other screening measures. The signs and symptoms most often associated with thyroid storm include hyperthermia, tachycardia, tachydysrhythmias, central nervous system symptoms (e.g., psychosis, altered mental state), and rhabdomyolysis. Although thyrotoxic crisis can occur intraoperatively, the onset more frequently occurs 6 to 18 hours postoperatively. Precipitating factors include infection, surgery, diabetic ketoacidosis, congestive heart failure, pregnancy, and extreme physiologic stress. Without treatment, thyroid storm can be fatal, and mortality ranges from 10% to 75%.

SIGNS AND SYMPTOMS

Respiratory

- Rales caused by congestive heart failure
- Shortness of breath

Cardiovascular

- Chest pain
- Diaphoresis
- Dilated cardiomyopathy
- Dysrhythmias
- Hypertension
- Orthostatic hypotension
- Tachycardia

Other considerations

- Agitation, anxiety, delirium
- Elevated blood glucose
- Elevated hematocrit
- Exophthalmos
- Goiter
- Headaches
- Hyperthermia
- Nausea
- Seizures

DIFFERENTIAL DIAGNOSIS

Neurologic

- Intracranial lesions
- Neuroleptic malignant syndrome

Respiratory

- Endobronchial intubation/endotracheal tube stimulating the carina
- Hypercarbia
- Hypoxia

Cardiovascular

- Cardiac dysrhythmias
- Congestive heart failure
- Hypertensive crises
- Myocardial infarction
- Untreated essential hypertension

Renal

• Acute renal dysfunction

Endocrine

• Carcinoid syndrome
• Hypermetabolic syndromes (e.g., neuroleptic malignant syndrome)

Pharmacologic

• Central anticholinergic syndrome (e.g., atropine overdose)
• Monoamine oxidase inhibitors
• Opioid and/or alcohol withdrawal
• Psychotropic medications which can cause neuroleptic malignant syndrome (e.g., haloperidol, chlorpromazine, metoclopramide, lithium)
• Sympathomimetics
    1. Drug misuse (e.g., cocaine, methamphetamine)
    2. Therapeutic medications (e.g., epinephrine)

Other considerations

• Malignant hyperthermia
• Inadequate depth of anesthesia during surgical stimulation
• Preeclampsia/eclampsia
• Serotonin syndrome

Diagnostic tests

• Thyroid function tests: thyroxine (T4)
• Triiodothyronine (T3)
• Thyroid-stimulating hormone

Suggested Readings

• Karlet M. The endocrine system and anesthesia. In: Elisha S, Heiner JS, Nagelhout JJ, eds. *Nurse Anesthesia*. 7th ed. St. Louis: Elsevier; 2023:851-894.
• Shahid M, Kiran Z, Sarfraz A, Hasan SM, Adnan SM, Baloch AA. Presentations and outcomes of thyroid storm. *J Coll Physicians Surg Pak*. 2020;30(3):330-331.
• Strowd SM, Majewski MB, Asteris J. Malignant hyperthermia versus thyroid storm in a patient with symptomatic Grave's disease: a case report. *A A Pract*. 2018;10(5):97-99.
• Sullivan K, Helgeson J, McGowan A. COVID-19 associated thyroid storm: a case report. *Clin Pract Cases Emerg Med*. 2021;5(4):412-414.
• Ylli D, Klubo-Gwiezdzinska J, Wartofsky L. Thyroid emergencies. *Pol Arch Intern Med*. 2019;129(7-8):526-534.

CHAPTER 34   Disseminated Intravascular Coagulation (DIC)

MANAGEMENT

PRIMARY ACTIONS

- Treat underlying pathological state
- Goal-directed crystalloid, colloid, factor concentrates, and blood product component therapy (e.g., administration based on clinical and laboratory assessment)
- Avoid lethal triad: acidosis, hypothermia, and coagulopathy

SECONDARY ACTIONS

- Supportive measures, as necessary (see "Medications")
  1. Airway management and mechanical ventilation
  2. Invasive monitoring (e.g., arterial, central venous catheter)
  3. Monitor acid-base, fluid, and electrolyte balance
- Large-bore peripheral or central venous access
- Massive transfusion protocol
  1. Activate goal-directed massive transfusion protocol. For example, 4 units packed red blood cells + 4 units fresh frozen plasma + 1 pooled platelet unit (e.g., equal to 4-6 individual units)
  2. Adjunctive therapies as indicated (see "Medications")
  3. Autologous blood cell salvage and autotransfusion

MEDICATIONS

- Antibiotics, as appropriate
- Recombinant Factor VIIa 70 to 90 mcg/kg/dose IV, every 2-3 hours until hemostasis is achieved
- Antifibrinolytic (only for the hyperfibrinolytic state, otherwise contraindicated)
  - Aminocaproic acid 4-5 grams IV loading dose given over 1 hour, then 1 gram/h infusion for 8 hours and/or,
  - Tranexamic acid 10-30 mg/kg IV given over 10-30 minutes
- Vasopressor(s) to maintain MAP > 65 mm Hg:
  - Ephedrine 5-10 mg IV bolus and/or,
  - Phenylephrine 50-100 mcg IV bolus, 0.1-0.5 mcg/kg/min infusion and/or,
  - Epinephrine 10-100 mcg IV bolus, 0.1-0.5 mcg/kg/min infusion and/or,
  - Dopamine 5-20 mcg/kg/min IV infusion and/or,
  - Norepinephrine 5-10 mcg IV bolus, 0.1-0.5 mcg/kg/min infusion and/or,
  - Vasopressin 1-4 Unit IV bolus, 0.01-0.1 Units/min infusion

PHYSIOLOGY/PATHOPHYSIOLOGY

Disseminated intravascular coagulation (DIC) is a symptom of a primary pathological process. Conditions that predispose patients to DIC include (1) sepsis, (2) massive trauma and shock states, (3) obstetrical complications, (4) malignant disease, (5) vascular disease, (6) immune-mediated disorders, (7) systemic toxins, (9) primary organ failure, and (10) intravascular hemolysis. Therefore, treatment for DIC must focus on identifying and correcting the underlying pathological state.

In DIC, there is systemic inflammation, coagulation activation, and fibrinolysis. Clinical presentation of DIC may include thrombosis, hemorrhage, or both. Systemic activation of coagulation results in (1) intravascular deposition of fibrin, (2) thrombotic microangiopathy, (3) compromised blood supply to organs, and (4) multiorgan system failure. Activation of coagulation promotes the use and subsequent depletion of platelets and coagulation factors. This consumptive coagulopathy may induce severe bleeding from multiple sites.

SIGNS AND SYMPTOMS

Neurologic
- Altered level of consciousness
- Central nervous system abnormalities
- Signs of stroke with cerebral hemorrhage or thrombosis
  - Dizziness
  - Headache
  - Paralysis
  - Speech changes

Respiratory
- Decreased SpO_2
- Dyspnea
- Hypoxia

Cardiovascular
- Cardiac dysrhythmias
- Hemodynamic instability

Hematologic
- Hemorrhage
  1. Bleeding from mucous membranes and skin (e.g., petechiae, ecchymosis)

    2. Bleeding from surgical sites, wounds, catheters, invasive monitor sites, venipuncture sites, or mucosal surfaces

    3. Bruising

- Thrombosis
    1. Peripheral acrocyanosis (bluish discoloration of extremities)
    2. Pregangrenous changes to peripheral tissue (e.g., hands, feet, genitalia, nose)
    3. Purpura fulminans
    4. Thromboembolism
- Laboratory abnormalities
    1. Elevated fibrin degradation products (e.g., D-dimer immunoassay)
    2. Moderate to severe hypofibrinogenemia
    3. Moderate to severe thrombocytopenia
    4. Prolonged clotting time (e.g., prothrombin time, activated partial thromboplastin time)

Other considerations

- Fever
- Multiorgan system failure
    1. Elevated serum markers (e.g., hepatic, renal, cardiac)

DIFFERENTIAL DIAGNOSIS

Neurologic

- Stroke
- Traumatic brain injury

Respiratory

- Acute respiratory distress syndrome

Cardiovascular

- Fat embolism
- Hypovolemia
- Vascular disease
    1. Kasabach-Merritt syndrome (e.g., giant hemangioma)
    2. Large-vessel aneurysm (e.g., aortic aneurysm)

Hematologic

- Hemolytic transfusion reaction
- Heparin-induced thrombocytopenia
- Massive transfusion
- Thrombotic microangiopathy
- Thrombotic thrombocytopenic purpura

Gastrointestinal

• Fulminant hepatic failure

Pharmacologic

• Drug misuse (e.g., methamphetamine overdose)

Other considerations

• Immune-mediated disorders
    1. Adult Still disease
    2. Allergic reactions
    3. Lupus erythematosus
    4. Transplant rejection
• Malignant disease
    1. Cytotoxic chemotherapy
    2. Myeloproliferative malignancy (e.g., acute promyelocytic leukemia)
    3. Pancreatic carcinoma
    4. Solid tumors (e.g., metastatic adenocarcinoma)
    5. Trousseau syndrome (e.g., chronic compensated DIC)
    6. Tumor lysis syndrome
• Massive trauma and shock states
    1. Extensive burns
• Obstetrical complications
    1. Amniotic fluid embolism
    2. HELLP syndrome (e.g., hemolysis, elevated liver function tests, low platelets)
    3. Placenta previa
    4. Placental abruption
    5. Retained fetus and/or products of conception syndrome
    6. Septic miscarriage or abortion
• Sepsis
    1. Fungal
    2. Gram-negative and gram-positive bacteria
    3. Helminthic
    4. Malaria
    5. Protozoan
    6. Rocky Mountain spotted fever
    7. Viral illnesses
• Systemic toxins
    1. Snake venom

Diagnostic tests

• Arterial blood gas
• Complete blood count
• D-dimer

- Fibrinogen
- Functional hemodynamic monitoring (e.g., stroke volume variation, pulse pressure variation, Pleth variability index)
- Prothrombin time, activated partial thromboplastin time, activated clotting time
- Serum electrolyte test(s): sodium, potassium, calcium, magnesium
- Thromboelastography (TEG) or rotational thromboelastometry (ROTEM)
- Type and screen/crossmatch

Suggested Readings

- Brazzel C. Thromboelastography-guided transfusion therapy in the trauma patient. *AANA J.* 2013;81(2):127-132.
- Collins S, MacIntyre C, Hewer I. Thromboelastography: clinical application, interpretation, and transfusion management. *AANA J.* 2016;84(2):129-134.
- Franco JA, Gabot MH. Hematology and anesthesia. In: Elisha S, Heiner JS, Nagelhout JJ, eds. *Nurse Anesthesia.* 7th ed. St. Louis: Elsevier; 2023:895-916.
- Squizzato A, Hunt BJ, Kinasewitz GT, et al. Supportive management strategies for disseminated intravascular coagulation. An international consensus. *Thromb Haemost.* 2016;115(5): 896-904. doi:10.1160/TH15-09-0740.

CHAPTER 35   Hemoglobinopathies

MANAGEMENT

PRIMARY ACTIONS

- Identify the type of hemoglobinopathy (e.g., carboxyhemoglobin, methemoglobin, sickle cell crisis)
- Stop triggering agents
- Administer 100% FiO_2 (e.g., high-flow oxygen, nonrebreathing face mask)
- Hyperbaric oxygen, if available
- Avoid lethal triad: acidosis, hypothermia, and coagulopathy
- See Table 35-1 for management of specific hemoglobinopathies

SECONDARY ACTIONS

- Supportive measures as necessary (see "Medications")
  1. Airway management and mechanical ventilation
  2. Invasive monitoring (e.g., arterial line, central venous pressure)
  3. Monitor acid-base, fluid, and electrolyte balance
  4. Large-bore peripheral IV or central venous access

MEDICATIONS

For treatment of methemoglobinemia:

- Methylene blue 1-2 mg/kg IV infusion, maximum dose 100 mg, may repeat dose after 1 hour if methemoglobin level remains $> 30\%$ or symptoms persist
- Ascorbic acid 1-10 grams IV infusion, every 6 hours until methemoglobin levels normalize (for patients with G6PD deficiency or taking serotonergic medication)
- Vasopressor(s) to maintain MAP > 65 mm Hg:
  - Ephedrine 5-10 mg IV bolus and/or,
  - Phenylephrine 50-100 mcg IV bolus, 0.1-0.5 mcg/kg/min infusion and/or,
  - Epinephrine 10-100 mcg IV bolus, 0.1-0.5 mcg/kg/min infusion and/or,
  - Dopamine 5-20 mcg/kg/min IV infusion and/or,
  - Norepinephrine 5-10 mcg IV bolus, 0.1-0.5 mcg/kg/min infusion and/or,
  - Vasopressin 1-4 Unit IV bolus, 0.01-0.1 Units/min infusion

PHYSIOLOGY AND PATHOPHYSIOLOGY

Hemoglobinopathies include carboxyhemoglobin (COHb), methemoglobin (MetHb), and sickle cell crisis (SCC). Hemoglobinopathies decrease (1) the oxygen-carrying capacity of red blood cells, (2) the transport and use of oxygen, and (3) cause end-organ ischemia. As measured by SpO_2, the oxygen saturation of

Table 35-1 Characteristics of specific hemoglobinopathies

	TRIGGERING AGENTS	SIGNS AND SYMPTOMS	MANAGEMENT

Carboxyhemoglobin (COHb)	• Smoke inhalation
	• Poorly functioning heating systems
	• Use of fuel-burning devices and/or motor vehicles with improper ventilation
	• Volatile anesthetic degradation (particularly with desiccated carbon dioxide absorbent granules and/or low-flow anesthesia)
		• COHb levels > 5%
		• Headache (most common)
		• Dizziness and weakness
		• Nausea/vomiting
		• Altered level of consciousness
		• Chest pain
		• Respiratory distress
			• Remove CO source
			• Administer 100% FiO_2 (e.g., high-flow oxygen, nonbreathing face mask)
			• Hyperbaric oxygen for:
			  1. CO level > 25%
			  2. CO level > 20% in a pregnant patient
			  3. Loss of consciousness
			  4. Severe metabolic acidosis (pH < 7.1)
			  5. Evidence of end-organ ischemia
			• Mechanical ventilation, as necessary
			• Supportive measures
			• Psychiatric evaluation for intentional poisoning

Methemoglobin (MetHb)	• Ingested medication (e.g., dapsone, antimalarial) • Local anesthetics (e.g., benzocaine, lidocaine, prilocaine) • Nitrates or nitrites (e.g., nitroglycerine, nitroprusside) • Inhaled nitric oxide • Metoclopramide • Methylene blue (high doses)	• MetHb levels > 5% • Cyanosis • Dyspnea • Neurological symptoms from headache to coma • Respiratory depression	• Remove triggering agent • Administer 100% FiO_2 (e.g., high-flow oxygen, nonbreathing face mask) • Hyperbaric oxygen • Methylene blue (see "Medications") • Ascorbic acid (see "Medications") • Mechanical ventilation, as necessary • Supportive measures • Consider transfusion or exchange transfusion

Continued

Table 35-1 Characteristics of specific hemoglobinopathies—cont'd

	TRIGGERING AGENTS	SIGNS AND SYMPTOMS	MANAGEMENT
Sickle cell crisis (SCC)	• Cold environment • Weather fluctuations (e.g., wind, low humidity) • Dehydration • Stress • Alcohol	• Infection • Hemolytic anemia • Vaso-occlusion (e.g., acute/chronic pain, tissue ischemia, infarction)	• Remove triggering agent • Administer 100% FiO_2 (e.g., high-flow oxygen, nonbreathing face mask) • Hyperbaric oxygen • Active warming measures (e.g., forced-air convective warmer, warmed fluids) • Maintain adequate hydration • Multimodal pain management using opioid and nonopioid analgesics (e.g., acetaminophen, nonsteroidal anti-inflammatory drugs, ketamine, gabapentin) • Antibiotics, as necessary • Supportive measures • Consider blood product transfusion

CO, carbon monoxide

hemoglobin is inaccurate with high COHb and MetHb levels. What results is a consistent overestimation of the SpO_2 oxygen saturation. In these cases, practitioners should use arterial blood gas and/or co-oximetry to guide diagnosis and treatment.

Carbon monoxide (CO) has an affinity for hemoglobin 200 times greater than oxygen. Accidental or intentional exposure to high concentrations of CO leads to preferential binding of CO to hemoglobin forming COHb. CO causes a left shift in the oxyhemoglobin dissociation curve, decreasing the ability of hemoglobin to release bound oxygen. Furthermore, CO impairs oxygen use and oxidative phosphorylation at the cellular level. Treatment of CO poisoning focuses on providing supplemental inspired oxygen at 100% FiO_2 because this decreases the half-life of CO from 4 hours with room air to 60 to 90 minutes.

MetHb is formed by the oxidation of hemoglobin and alteration of its heme iron configuration from a ferrous (Fe^{2+}) to ferric (Fe^{3+}) state. Congenital or acquired MetHb prevents oxygen binding, causes a left shift in the oxyhemoglobin dissociation curve, and decreases oxygen tissue delivery. Treatment of MetHb includes methylene blue. Methylene blue should be used with caution in patients with a glucose-6-phosphate dehydrogenase (G6PD) deficiency or receiving serotonergic medications because it can precipitate hemolysis or serotonin syndrome. In these cases, ascorbic acid is an alternative treatment.

Sickle cell anemia is caused by a point mutation in the beta-globin gene and results in the production of hemoglobin S (HbS). When HbS is exposed to low oxygen tension it forms elongated crystals, this results in distortion of the cell membrane and the red blood cell (RBC) becomes sickle shaped. The RBCs are unable to pass through small capillaries and rupture the cell membranes leading to sickle cell anemia. Signs and symptoms of sickle cell crisis (SCC) (e.g., vaso-occlusive crisis) include painful episodes, tissue ischemia, and end-organ infarction. SCC is can be caused by low oxygen tension, hypoxia, acidosis, illness, stress, and dehydration. Prevention and treatment of acute SCC includes maintaining normothermia, ensuring adequate hydration, supplemental oxygen, and providing multimodal analgesia.

SIGNS AND SYMPTOMS
Neurologic

- Coma
- Confusion
- Delayed neurologic sequelae (e.g., cognitive deficits, personality changes, movement disorders, focal neurological deficits)
- Encephalopathy

- Headache
- Lightheadedness
- Loss of consciousness/syncope
- Proliferative retinopathy
- Seizures
- Stroke (e.g., hemorrhagic, ischemic)
- Transient ischemic attack

Respiratory

- Cor pulmonale
- Cyanosis
- Dyspnea
- Hypoxia
- Pulmonary edema
- Pulmonary fibrosis
- Pulmonary infarction
- Respiratory depression

Cardiovascular

- Cardiomegaly
- Cardiomyopathy with diastolic dysfunction
- Chest pain
- Dysrhythmia
- Myocardial ischemia/infarction
- Vaso-occlusive pain
- Venous thromboembolism
- Ventricular arrhythmias

Musculoskeletal

- Bone marrow infarcts
- Growth impairment
- Osteomyelitis

Hematological

- Anemia (e.g., megaloblastic, aplastic)
- Hyperhemolytic crisis
- Leukocytosis
- Pancytopenia
- Disseminated intravascular coagulation
- Splenic or hepatic crisis (e.g., sequestration, infarction)

Renal

- Hematuria
- Renal infarction/failure

Other considerations

- "Cherry red" lips and skin
- Chronic leg ulcers
- Dactylitis (acute pain in the hands or feet)
- Fatigue/malaise
- Fever
- Infection (e.g., bacteremia, meningitis, pulmonary)
- Jaundice
- Lactic/metabolic acidosis
- Nausea/vomiting
- Priapism

DIFFERENTIAL DIAGNOSIS

Neurological

- Intracranial hemorrhage
- Ischemic encephalopathy
- Seizures
- Stroke

Respiratory

- Acute respiratory distress syndrome
- Airway obstruction
- Bronchospasm
- Obstructive sleep apnea
- Pneumonia
- Pneumothorax
- Pulmonary edema
- Pulmonary embolism
- Pulmonary hypertension

Cardiovascular

- Acute chest/coronary syndrome
- Cardiogenic shock
- Congestive heart failure
- Deep vein thrombosis
- Myocardial ischemia

Musculoskeletal

- Acute synovitis with avascular necrosis
- Arthritis
- Neuromuscular disorders (e.g., muscular dystrophy)
- Osteoporosis

Hematological

- Acute viral syndrome
- Hemolytic transfusion reaction
- Polycythemia
- Sulfhemoglobinemia
- Transfusion iron overload

Endocrine

- Severe hypoglycemia

Other considerations

- Acute papillary necrosis
- Acute surgery of the abdomen (e.g., cholecystitis)
- Gout
- Opioid withdrawal
- Sepsis
- Sudden death syndrome

Diagnostic tests

- Arterial blood gas (e.g., carboxyhemoglobin, methemoglobin)
- Blood chemistry panel
- Cardiac biomarkers (e.g., cardiac troponin, creatinine kinase-MB, myoglobin)
- Chest radiograph
- Complete blood count
- Co-oximetry
- Electrocardiogram
- Imaging studies of the head (e.g., computed tomography, magnetic resonance imaging, positron emission tomography)
- Liver function tests
- Pregnancy test
- Toxicology screen (e.g., cyanide)

Suggested Readings

- Harbin KR, Norris TE. Anesthetic management of patients with major burn injury. *AANA J.* 2012;80(6):430-439.
- Khurmi N, Gorlin A, Misra L. Perioperative considerations for patients with sickle cell disease: a narrative review. *Can J Anaesth.* 2017;64(8):860-869. doi:10.1007/s12630-017-0883-3.
- Kulcke A, Feiner J, Menn I, Holmer A, Hayoz J, Bickler P. The accuracy of pulse spectroscopy for detecting hypoxemia and coexisting methemoglobin or carboxyhemoglobin. *Anesth Analg.* 2016;122(6):1856-1865. doi:10.1213/ANE.0000000000001219.
- Levy RJ. Anesthesia-related carbon monoxide exposure: toxicity and potential therapy. *Anesth Analg.* 2016;123(3):670-681. doi:10.1213/ANE.0000000000001461.

CHAPTER 36　Transfusion-Related Emergencies

MANAGEMENT

PRIMARY ACTIONS

- Identify the type of transfusion-related emergency (e.g., TRALI, TACO, AHTR)
- Stop blood product transfusion immediately
- Provide supplemental oxygen
- Noninvasive supportive ventilation, such as continuous positive airway pressure (CPAP) or bilevel positive airway pressure (BiPAP) as necessary
- Avoid lethal triad: acidosis, hypothermia, and coagulopathy

SECONDARY ACTIONS

- See Table 36-1 for management of specific transfusion-related emergencies
- Supportive measures as necessary (see "Medications")
- Airway management and mechanical ventilation
  1. Lung protective tidal volume of 6-8 mL/kg
  2. Peak inspiratory pressure less than 30 cmH$_2$O to prevent volutrauma and barotrauma
  3. Positive end-expiratory pressure of 5-10 cmH$_2$O to promote alveolar recruitment
- Invasive monitoring (e.g., arterial pressure, central venous pressure)
- Monitor acid-base, fluid, and electrolyte balance
- Sequester suspected blood products, report the emergency to the blood bank, and initiate institution-specific transfusion-related reaction protocol

MEDICATIONS

- Furosemide 20-40 mg IV bolus
- Vasopressor(s) to maintain MAP > 65 mm/Hg:
  - Ephedrine 5-10 mg IV bolus and or,
  - Phenylephrine 50-100 mcg IV bolus, 0.1-0.5 mcg/kg/min infusion and/or,
  - Epinephrine 10-100 mcg IV bolus, 0.1-0.5 mcg/kg/min infusion and/or,
  - Dopamine 5-20 mcg/kg/min IV infusion and/or,
  - Norepinephrine 5-10 mcg IV bolus, 0.1-0.5 mcg/kg/min infusion and/or,
  - Vasopressin 1-4 Unit IV bolus, 0.01-0.1 Units/min infusion

Table 36-1 Characteristics of transfusion-related emergencies

	SIGNS AND SYMPTOMS	ONSET AFTER START OF BLOOD PRODUCT ADMINISTRATION	MANAGEMENT
Transfusion-related acute lung injury (TRALI)	• New-onset acute respiratory distress syndrome: 1. Hypoxemia: oxygen saturation is ≤ 90% on room air or a PaO_2/FiO_2 ratio ≤ 300 mm Hg 2. Abnormal chest radiograph (e.g., bilateral pulmonary infiltrates) • Noncardiogenic pulmonary edema	1-2 h, up to 6 h	• Discontinue blood product administration • Supplemental oxygen • CPAP or BiPAP • Mechanical ventilation as necessary • Supportive measures • Initiation of the institution-specific transfusion-related reaction protocol
Transfusion-associated circulatory overload (TACO)	• New onset or exacerbation of three or more of the following criteria: 1. Acute respiratory distress syndrome 2. Pulmonary edema as evidenced on physical examination or chest radiograph 3. Elevated brain natriuretic protein (BNP) or N-terminal prohormone BNP (NT-pro BNP) 4. Other unexplained cardiovascular changes (e.g., increased central venous pressure) • Cardiogenic (hydrostatic) pulmonary edema	1-2 h, up to 12 h	• Discontinue blood product administration • Supplemental oxygen • CPAP or BiPAP • Fluid mobilization using diuretics (see "Medications") • Mechanical ventilation as necessary • Supportive measures • Initiation of the institution-specific transfusion-related reaction protocol

| Acute hemolytic transfusion reaction (AHTR) | • Classic triad
  1. Fever
  2. Flank or back pain
  3. Red or brown-colored urine (e.g., hemo-
     globinuria, hematuria)
• Other symptoms:
  1. Chills
  2. DIC
  3. Hypotension
  4. Hemoglobinemia
  5. Oliguria | 1-2 h, up to 24 h | • Discontinue blood product
  administration
• Supplemental oxygen
• CPAP or BiPAP
• Mechanical ventilation as necessary
• Supportive measures
• Aggressive hydration
• Diuretics (see "Medications")
• Initation of the institution-specific
  transfusion-related reaction protocol |

AHTR, acute hemolytic transfusion reaction; *BiPAP*, bilevel positive airway pressure; *CPAP*, continuous postitive airway pressure; *DIC*, disseminated intravascular coagulation; *TACO*, transfusion-associated circulatory overload; *TRALI*, transfusion-related acute lung injury

PHYSIOLOGY/PATHOPHYSIOLOGY

Transfusion-related emergencies (TREs) are classified as transfusion-related acute lung injury (TRALI), transfusion-associated circulatory overload (TACO), and acute hemolytic transfusion reaction (AHTR). TREs are the leading cause of transfusion-related morbidity and mortality. The development of TREs is associated with the administration of blood products, including whole blood, packed red blood cells, fresh-frozen plasma, platelet products, cryoprecipitate, intravenous immunoglobulin, and stem cell preparations. TREs are immune-mediated processes. Primary management for TREs focuses on the immediate discontinuation of the blood product transfusion, supportive measures, and initiating institution-specific transfusion-related reaction protocols.

TRALI is a two-stage process. First, patient-related risk factors (e.g., smoking, inflammation, infection) recruit neutrophils into the lungs. Second, pathogenic transfusion antibodies or biological response modifiers from blood products activate primed neutrophils causing alveolar-capillary damage, increased pulmonary capillary permeability, and noncardiogenic pulmonary edema.

TACO is also a two-staged immune response. TACO occurs when patient-related risk factors (such as cardiac or renal impairment) act as immunological priming mechanisms. Subsequently, suboptimal fluid management or other components within the transfused product causes an immune-mediated response, acute respiratory distress, and cardiogenic (hydrostatic) pulmonary edema.

In contrast, AHTR is the result of a clerical error (e.g., mislabeling a collection sample) or an administrative error (e.g., transfusion of packed red blood cells to the wrong patient). These errors lead to the transfusion of ABO-incompatible packed red blood cells. Subsequent complement cascade activation leads to antigen-antibody complexes that act against the allogeneic red blood cell antigen and cause intravascular hemolysis. The classic triad of acute hemolytic transfusion reaction (AHTR) includes (1) fever, (2) flank or back pain, and (3) red or brown-colored urine (e.g., hemoglobinuria, hematuria). AHTR can progress to mixed shock states and disseminated intravascular coagulation.

SIGNS AND SYMPTOMS

Respiratory

- Acute respiratory distress (e.g., dyspnea, orthopnea, cough, tachypnea, rales)
- Cardiogenic pulmonary edema

- Decreased lung compliance
- Decreased ratio of arterial oxygen partial pressure to the fraction of inspired oxygen
- Hypoxemia
  1. Clinical signs and symptoms of hypoxia (e.g., cyanosis)
  2. $PaO_2 < 60$ mm Hg on room air
  3. PaO_2 to FiO_2 ratio ≤ 300
  4. $SpO_2 < 90\%$ on room air
- Noncardiogenic pulmonary edema
- Pulmonary infiltrates

Cardiovascular

- Hypertension
- Hypotension
- Tachycardia

Hematologic

- Laboratory findings
  1. Anemia
  2. Decreased fibrinogen
  3. Decreased haptoglobin
  4. Elevated bilirubin
  5. Leukopenia
  6. Neutropenia
  7. Monocytopenia
  8. Hypocomplementemia
  9. Demonstration of human leukocyte antigen (HLA) class I or class II
  10. Matching leukocyte antibody-antigen in the donor-recipient

Other considerations

- Acute onset (e.g., within 24 hours of transfusion)
- Disseminated intravascular coagulation (DIC)
- Evidence of positive fluid balance
- Fever and/or chills
- Flank pain
- Hemoglobinemia
- No existing acute lung injury before transfusion
- No relationship to alternative risk factors for acute lung injury
- Rash and/or urticaria
- Red or brown-colored urine (e.g., hemoglobinuria, hematuria)

DIFFERENTIAL DIAGNOSIS

Neurologic

- Neurogenic pulmonary edema

Respiratory

- Acute respiratory distress syndrome (ARDS)
- Aspiration (e.g., gastric contents and near-drowning)
- Inhalation injury (e.g., thermal or caustic chemicals)
- Pneumonia
- Reexpansion pulmonary edema (e.g., postthoracic surgery requiring one-lung ventilation)

Cardiovascular

- Cardiogenic problems with increased pulmonary capillary pressure
  1. Acute or chronic valvular disease
  2. Cardiac dysrhythmias
  3. Cardiomyopathy
  4. Congestive heart failure
  5. Constrictive pericarditis
  6. Left-ventricular failure
  7. Myocardial infarction or ischemia
  8. Pericardial tamponade
- Myocardial infarction
- Noncardiogenic increased pulmonary capillary pressure
  1. Circulatory volume overload (e.g., fluid overload)
  2. Negative pressure pulmonary edema
  3. Pulmonary embolism
- Reperfusion pulmonary edema (e.g., postpulmonary thrombectomy, transplantation, or cardiopulmonary bypass)
- Shock states

Hematologic

- Disseminated intravascular coagulation (DIC)
- Hypoalbuminemia
- Immune-mediated reaction

Pharmacologic

- Drug overdose

Other considerations

- Amniotic fluid embolism
- Angioedema
- Anaphylaxis
- Fat embolus
- High-altitude pulmonary edema
- Immersion pulmonary edema
- Infectious disease
- Ischemia-reperfusion injury

- Preeclampsia
- Renal failure
- Systemic inflammatory response syndrome (e.g., sepsis)

Diagnostic tests

- Arterial blood gas
- Brain natriuretic peptide
- Complete blood count
- Chest radiograph
- Echocardiography (e.g., transthoracic, transesophageal)
- Tryptase
- Type and screen/crossmatch

Suggested Readings

- McVey MJ, Kapur R, Cserti-Gazdewich C, Semple JW, Karkouti K, Kuebler WM. Transfusion-related acute lung injury in the perioperative patient. *Anesthesiology*. 2019;131(3):693-715. doi: 10.1097/ALN.0000000000002687.
- Semple JW, Rebetz J, Kapur R. Transfusion-associated circulatory overload and transfusion-related acute lung injury. *Blood*. 2019;133(17):1840-1853. doi:10.1182/blood-2018-10-860809.
- Yazer MH, Waters JH, Spinella PC. Use of uncrossmatched erythrocytes in emergency bleeding situations. *Anesthesiology*. 2018;128(3):650-656. doi:10.1097/ALN.0000000000002037.

CHAPTER 37   Local Anesthetic Systemic Toxicity (LAST)

MANAGEMENT

PRIMARY ACTIONS

If mild to moderate signs and symptoms of LAST occur:
- Stop local anesthetic (LA) injection
- Administer 100% oxygen
- Assess airway, breathing, and circulation
- Administer medications such as midazolam or propofol to increase the seizure threshold

If severe signs and symptoms of LAST occur and/or the patient condition deteriorates:
- Call for help
- Stop LA injection
- Assess adequacy of/breathing
  1. Maintain and secure a patent airway
  2. Ensure adequate oxygenation and ventilation to prevent hypoxia, hypercarbia, acidosis, and ion trapping
- Assess circulation
  1. Definitive treatment is Intralipid 20% IV (see "Medications")
  2. Administer IV fluid bolus
  3. Administer medications such as midazolam or propofol to increase the seizure threshold
  4. Neuromuscular blockade for persistent tonic-clonic seizure activity
  5. Treat hypotension (see "Medications")
  6. For severe or sustained bradycardia, administer atropine (see "Medications")

SECONDARY ACTIONS

- Perform ACLS or PALS per American Heart Association protocol
- Consider cardiopulmonary bypass

MEDICATIONS

- *Fat emulsion (Intralipid) 20%*
  - Patients > 70 kg, administer Intralipid 20% 100 mL IV bolus over 2-3 minutes, then 0.25 mL/kg/min infusion
  - Patients < 70 kg, administer Intralipid 20% 1.5 mL/kg IV bolus, then 0.25 mL/kg/min infusion

- Repeat Intralipid bolus dose every 5 minutes (maximum of 3 bolus doses), and increase the infusion to 0.5 mL/kg/min for persistent hemodynamic instability
- Maximum intralipid total dose is 12 mL/kg IV
- Vasopressor(s) to maintain MAP > 65 mm Hg:
  - Ephedrine 5-10 mg IV bolus and/or,
  - Phenylephrine 50-100 mcg IV bolus, 0.1-0.5 mcg/kg/min infusion and/or,
  - Epinephrine 10-100 mcg IV bolus, 0.1-0.5 mcg/kg/min infusion and/or,
  - Dopamine 5-20 mcg/kg/min IV infusion and/or,
  - Norepinephrine 5-10 mcg bolus, 0.1-0.5 mcg/kg/min infusion and/or,
  - Vasopressin 1-4 Unit bolus, 0.01-0.1 Units/min infusion
- Atropine 0.5-1.0 mg IV bolus

PHYSIOLOGY AND PATHOPHYSIOLOGY

Local anesthetic (LA) medications attenuate the propagation of action potentials along nerves by inhibiting sodium channels and depolarization. As a result, the motor, sensory, and vascular sympathetic nervous system tone is inhibited. Compared with the heart, the brain is more sensitive to the effects of elevated plasma concentrations of LA. This explains why, as the LA concentration increases, manifestations begin with mild to moderate neurologic signs and symptoms, then progress to severe neurologic signs, and finally, cardiotoxicity ensues. Hypoxia, hypercarbia, and acidosis potentiate ion trapping and cardiotoxicity. The suspected causes of cardiotoxicity include LA blockade of cardiac sodium, potassium, and calcium channels and cardiomyocyte mitochondrial inhibition. Due to its high potency and protein binding, bupivacaine is the LA most often implicated in cases of cardiac arrest caused by LAST. LAST is dependent on multiple factors, including:
1. Accidental injection of the LA into an artery or vein
2. Addition of epinephrine, which slows the LA absorption into plasma
3. Potency of the LA (greater potency will cause toxicity at lower plasma concentrations)
4. Speed of absorption of the LA into plasma
5. The ability of the patient to metabolize and excrete the LA
6. Total LA plasma concentration (mg/kg dose)

Prevention of LA toxicity is best accomplished by:
1. Addition of epinephrine into the LA solution tests for intravascular injection (as indicated by increased heart rate) and slows LA absorption into plasma
2. Aspiration before injection of LA to check for blood and/or cerebrospinal fluid (high spinal)

3. Calculation and communication of the toxic dose based on the kilogram weight of the patient before LA administration by the anesthesia provider (e.g., the total dose of topical, intravenous, regional, neuraxial anesthesia) and/or the surgeon (e.g., surgical site infiltration, intra-articular injection)
4. Consistent verbal communication with the patient to assess the level of consciousness and other signs and symptoms associated with neurologic LAST
5. Injection of LA in 3-5 mL increments for epidural, fascial plane, or peripheral nerve blocks
6. Maintaining injection pressures for peripheral nerve blocks < 20 psi
7. Use of ultrasound for fascial plane and peripheral nerve blocks

SIGNS AND SYMPTOMS

Mild to moderate neurologic manifestations-of LA toxicity

- Altered level of consciousness
- Circumoral/tongue numbness
- Diplopia
- Disorientation
- Lightheadedness
- Metallic taste in the mouth
- Muscular twitching
- Tinnitus

Severe neurologic manifestations of LA toxicity

- Coma
- Respiratory arrest
- Seizures
- Unconsciousness

Severe cardiac manifestations of LA toxicity

- Cardiac arrest
- Dysrhythmias
- Heart block
- Ventricular fibrillation
- Ventricular tachycardia

DIFFERENTIAL DIAGNOSIS

Neurologic

- Cerebrovascular accident
- Neurogenic shock from neuraxial anesthesia

- Pre-existing neurological disorders (e.g., seizure disorder, intracranial mass)

Respiratory

- Anxiety
- Hyperventilation
- Hypoxia

Cardiovascular

- See prior
- Myocardial ischemia/infarction
- Severe hypotension

Pharmacologic

- Local anesthetic overdose
- Regional anesthesia administration
- Sympathomimetic drug use (e.g., cocaine, methamphetamine)
- Total spinal/epidural blockade
- Vasovagal reaction

Other considerations

- Acidosis
- Anaphylaxis
- Eclampsia
- Hyponatremia (e.g., transurethral resection of the prostate syndrome)

Suggested Readings

- El-Boghdadly K, Pawa A, Chin KJ. Local anesthetic systemic toxicity: current perspectives. *Local Reg Anesth.* 2018;11:35-44.
- Gitman M, Fettiplace MR, Weinberg GL, Neal JM, Barrington MJ. Local anesthetic systemic toxicity: a narrative literature review and clinical update on prevention, diagnosis, and management. *Plast Reconstr Surg.* 2019;144(3):783-795.
- Nagelhout JJ. Local anesthetics. In: Elisha S, Heiner JS, Nagelhout JJ, eds. *Nurse Anesthesia.* 7th ed. St. Louis: Elsevier; 2023:118-150.
- Ok SH, Hong JM, Lee SH, Sohn JT. Lipid emulsion for treating local anesthetic systemic toxicity. *Int J Med Sci.* 2018;15(7): 713-722.
- Waldinger R, Weinberg G, Gitman M. Local anesthetic toxicity in the geriatric population. *Drugs Aging.* 2020;37(1):1-9.

CHAPTER 38   Malignant Hyperthermia (MH)

MANAGEMENT

PRIMARY ACTIONS

- Call for help, and obtain the malignant hyperthermia (MH) cart
- Notify the surgeon
- Stop any inhalation anesthetic agents and succinylcholine administration. Continue with non-MH triggering agents (e.g., propofol, nondepolarizing neuromuscular blocker)
- Maintain and secure a patent airway
- Provide adequate oxygenation and ventilation using a new breathing circuit and reservoir bag with high flow ($\geq$ 10 L/min) and 100% oxygen
- Apply activated charcoal filters to the inspiratory and expiratory limbs of the anesthesia gas machine
- Administer dantrolene (see "Medications")
- Cooling measures
  1. Forced air cooling
  2. Cooled IV fluids
  3. Intraperitoneal and/or intragastric lavage
- Consult the Malignant Hyperthermia Association of the United States (MHAUS) at 1-800-MH-HYPER (1-800-644-9737). Outside of North America: 001-209-417-3722

SECONDARY ACTIONS

- Invasive monitoring (arterial line) and obtain a second large-bore IV catheter
- IV fluid administration
- Increase minute ventilation
- Treat respiratory and metabolic acidosis
- Treat hyperkalemia if present (see "Medications")
- Treat dysrhythmias if present
- Obtain serial laboratory tests
  1. Arterial blood gas
  2. Electrolytes (particularly potassium)
  3. Coagulation panel
  4. Blood urea nitrogen and creatinine
  5. Creatinine kinase (CK)
- Perform ACLS or PALS per American Heart Association protocol

MEDICATIONS

- Dantrolene 2.5 mg/kg (actual body weight) IV bolus, repeat every 5 minutes up to 10 mg/kg until symptoms resolve

- *Dantrium and Revonto* formulations (20 mg/vial)
- Reconstitute with 60 mL sterile water
- For 70-kg patient, administer 9 vials (180 mg) IV bolus
- *Ryanodex* formulation (250 mg/vial)
- Reconstituted with 5 mL sterile water
- For 70-kg patient, administer 3.5 mL (175 mg) IV bolus

TREAT HYPERKALEMIA

- Regular insulin 5 Units IV bolus AND D50W (dextrose 25 g/ampule) 1-2 ampule IV bolus
- 10% calcium chloride 0.5-1 g IV over 10 minutes or 10% calcium gluconate 1-2 g IV over 2-5 minutes

TREAT METABOLIC ACIDOSIS

- 8.4% sodium bicarbonate 50 mEq (1 ampule) IV bolus over 5 minutes and/or 150 mEq in 1 L of D5W over 2-4 hours

PHYSIOLOGY AND PATHOPHYSIOLOGY

Malignant hyperthermia (MH) is an inherited genetic condition that predisposes intracellular skeletal ryanodine receptors (RYR1) to release excessive amounts of calcium when exposed to triggering agents such as inhalation anesthetics (sevoflurane, isoflurane, desflurane) and succinylcholine. Supraphysiologic calcium concentrations within skeletal myocytes cause voluntary and sustained skeletal muscle tetany. The increased oxygen demand and adenosine triphosphate requirements by skeletal muscles result in a hypermetabolic state that, if not reversed, leads to cellular hypoxia, acidosis, and death. The severity of the symptoms exhibited is proportional to the amount and rate of intracellular calcium released. Pathologic conditions predisposing patients to develop MH include central core disease and multiple types of muscular dystrophy (King-Denborough syndrome, myopathic disease, sarcoplasmic reticulum adenosine triphosphate deficiency).

Survivability after developing MH is dependent on prompt recognition and treatment with dantrolene, as well as the patient's preexisting medical history and functional status. Dantrolene begins to reverse the hypermetabolic effects associated with MH within 6 minutes. The mechanism of action of dantrolene causes desensitization of RYR1 receptors, which allows calcium to return to the sarcoplasmic reticulum, thus decreasing muscle contraction. Currently, the mortality rate associated with MH in the United States is approximately 5%.

SIGNS AND SYMPTOMS

Respiratory

- Decreased PaO_2
- Increased $PaCO_2$
- Unexplained increased $EtCO_2$ (most sensitive and specific initial clinical sign)

Cardiovascular

- Diaphoresis
- Dysrhythmias
- Hypertension
- Mottled and cyanotic skin
- Tachycardia (early sign but not specific)

Musculoskeletal

- Elevated CK
- Elevated urine and serum myoglobin
- Generalized muscle rigidity
- Masseter muscle spasm
- Rhabdomyolysis

Other considerations

- Disseminated intravascular coagulation
- Hyperkalemia
- Hyperthermia
- Myoglobinuria
- Respiratory and metabolic acidosis

DIFFERENTIAL DIAGNOSIS

Neurologic

- Hypothalamic lesions
- Neuroleptic malignant syndrome

Respiratory

- Endobronchial intubation and/or tube migration
- Hypercarbia
- Hypoventilation

Cardiovascular

- Shock states

Renal

- Acute renal dysfunction
- Myoglobinuria

Endocrine

- Carcinoid syndrome
- Hypermetabolic syndromes (e.g., pheochromocytoma, thyroid storm

Pharmacologic

- Central anticholinergic syndrome (e.g., atropine overdose)
- Monoamine oxidase inhibitors
- Opioid and/or alcohol withdrawal
- Psychotropic medications which can cause neuroleptic malignant syndrome (e.g., haloperidol, chlorpromazine, metoclopramide, lithium)
- Sympathomimetics
  1. Drug misuse (e.g., cocaine, methamphetamine)
  2. Therapeutic medications (e.g., epinephrine)

Other considerations

- Anaphylaxis
- CO_2 rebreathing (e.g., malfunctioning unidirectional valves)
- CO_2 absorption (e.g., laparoscopy or gastrointestinal endoscopy)
- Exhausted CO_2 granules (as evidenced by purple color change and/or elevated $FiCO_2$)
- Hyperthermia
- Hypovolemia
- Inadequate depth of anesthesia during surgical stimulation
- Sepsis
- Serotonin syndrome

Diagnostic tests

- Caffeine-halothane contracture test
- Genome sequencing

Suggested Readings

- Biesecker LG, Dirksen RT, Girard T, et al. Genomic screening for malignant hyperthermia susceptibility. *Anesthesiology.* 2020;133(6):1277-1282.
- Ellinas H, Albrecht MA. Malignant hyperthermia update. *Anesthesiol Clin.* 2020;38(1):165-181.
- Hopkins PM, Girard T, Dalay S, et al. Malignant hyperthermia 2020: Guideline from the Association of Anaesthetists. *Anaesthesia.* 2021;76(5):655-664.
- Karlet M. Musculoskeletal system anatomy, physiology, pathophysiology, and anesthesia management. In: Elisha S, Heiner

JS, Nagelhout JJ, eds. *Nurse Anesthesia*. 7th ed. St. Louis: Elsevier; 2023:826-850.
• White MD, Denborough MA. Dantrolene and calcium uptake by the sarcoplasmic reticulum of malignant hyperpyrexia-susceptible pigs. *Gen Pharmacol*. 1984;15(2):129-132.

CHAPTER 39 Neuroleptic Malignant Syndrome

MANAGEMENT

PRIMARY ACTIONS

- Discontinue dopamine antagonist (antipsychotic) therapy
  - Resume dopamine agonist in case of dopamine withdrawal (see "Medications")
  - Stop potential contributing agents (e.g., lithium, anticholinergic therapy, serotonergic agents)
- Obtain two large-bore IV access
- Place arterial line
- Maintain cardiovascular stability (MAP > 65 mm Hg)
  - Administer antiarrhythmic medications as indicated (see "Medications")
  - Provide cardiac pacing as needed
  - Manage hypertension (see "Medications")
- Provide mechanical ventilation as needed
- Rehydrate and maintain euvolemia
  - If *creatinine kinase* is elevated, administer IV fluid bolus and provide urine alkalinization
- Manage electrolyte abnormalities
- Treat hyperthermia
  - Cooling blankets, axillary ice packs, and if needed, ice water gastric lavage
  - Administer acetaminophen, ibuprofen, or aspirin

SECONDARY ACTIONS

- Manage agitation with benzodiazepines (see "Medications")
- Manage muscle rigidity with benzodiazepines or dantrolene (see "Medications")

MEDICATIONS

- Dopamine agonists
  - Bromocriptine 2.5 mg orally or via nasogastric tube every 6-8 hours
  - Amantadine 100-200 mg orally or via nasogastric tube every 12 hours
- Agitation:
  - Lorazepam 1-2 mg IV every 4-6 hours
  - Diazepam 10 mg IV every 8 hours
- Muscle rigidity
  - Dantrolene 1-2.5 mg/kg IV followed by 1 mg/kg IV infusion for 6 hours (maximum 10 mg/kg/d)
- Antiarrhythmic medications:

  - Amiodarone 150 mg IV over 10 minutes or,
  - Lidocaine 1-1.5 mg/kg IV
- Antihypertensive therapy:
  - Clonidine 0.2 mcg/kg/min infusion up to 0.5 mcg/kg/min or,
  - Sodium nitroprusside 0.3-0.5 mcg/kg/min (up to 2 mcg/kg/min) infusion
- Vasopressor(s) to maintain MAP > 65 mm Hg:
  - Ephedrine 5-10 mg IV bolus and/or,
  - Phenylephrine 50-100 mcg IV bolus, 0.1-0.5 mcg/kg/min infusion and/or,
  - Dopamine 5-20 mcg/kg/min IV infusion and/or,
  - Norepinephrine 5-10 mcg IV bolus, 0.1-0.5 mcg/kg/min infusion

PHYSIOLOGY AND PATHOPHYSIOLOGY

Neuroleptic malignant syndrome (NMS) is a life-threatening neurologic disease associated with the administration of dopamine antagonists such as antipsychotic (neuroleptic) medications, or rapid withdrawal of dopaminergic medications. Characteristics of NMS include mental status changes, hyperthermia (>38 °C), rigidity, significantly elevated creatine kinase (>1000 U/L) levels, and autonomic dysfunction. The neuroleptic medications that precipitate NMS are primarily first-generation antipsychotics such as haloperidol and fluphenazine. However, NMS can also occur after the administration of low-potency and second-generation antipsychotics such as chlorpromazine, clozapine, risperidone, and olanzapine. Antiemetics such as metoclopramide and promethazine have also been indicated with NMS (see Table 39-1 for medications associated with NMS).

Neuroleptic malignant syndrome can occur after a single antidopaminergic medication dose or even after many years of treatment. Risk factors include switching from one antipsychotic to another, rapid dose escalation, or parenteral (injection of infusion) administration. Other risk factors include certain psychiatric conditions, acute catatonia, extreme agitation, or simultaneous use of lithium, other psychotropic drugs, or substance abuse. Withdrawal from levodopa or dopamine agonist therapy in patients with Parkinson disease has also been associated with NMS.

The pathophysiology of NMS is not well understood. The primary theory focuses on the blockade of dopamine receptors within the central nervous and nigrostriatal systems. Dopamine receptor blockade in these areas can cause hyperpyrexia, rigidity, tremor, and autonomic dysfunction. It is possible that

Table 39-1 Medications associated with neuroleptic malignant syndrome*

Antipsychotic agents	Aripiprazole Chlorpromazine Clozapine Fluphenazine Haloperidol Olanzapine Paliperidone Perphenazine Quetiapine Risperidone Thioridazine Ziprasidone Amisulpride Zotepine
Antiemetic agents	Domperidone Droperidol Levosulpiride Metoclopramide Prochlorperazine Promethazine
Dopaminergic withdrawal	Levodopa Dopamine agonists Amantadine Tolcapone

*This is not a complete list because virtually every antipsychotic medication can cause neuroleptic malignant syndrome.

other neurotransmitters such as gamma aminobutyric acid, epinephrine, serotonin, and acetylcholine may also be involved. Alternative theories describe the following: (1) the disruption of the sympathetic nervous system that leads to an increase in metabolism and muscle tone along with unregulated vasomotor activity causing ineffective heat dissipation, labile blood pressures, and irregular heart rates; (2) excessive release of calcium from the sarcoplasmic reticulum of muscle cells caused by the administration of antipsychotic medications; and (3) a genetic component. Regardless of the mechanism, symptoms generally manifest over 1 to 3 days, and the diagnosis of NMS is made based on history and symptoms rather than any specific laboratory tests.

SIGNS AND SYMPTOMS

Neurologic

- Catatonia
- Coma
- Hyperthermia: > 38 °C (primary symptom)
- Mental status changes such as delirium or confusion (primary symptoms)

Respiratory

- Tachypnea

Cardiovascular

- Autonomic dysfunction (primary symptoms)
  - Diaphoresis
  - Dysrhythmias
  - Labile blood pressure
  - Sialorrhea
  - Skin pallor
  - Tachycardia
  - Urinary incontinence
- Electrocardiogram abnormalities
  - Prolonged PR, QRS, and QT intervals
  - ST and T-wave abnormalities

Musculoskeletal

TWO primary musculoskeletal signs of NMS include:
- Rigidity
- Significantly elevated creatinine kinase levels
  Other neuromuscular sign and symptoms include:
- Chorea (jerky, involuntary movements of shoulders, hands, hips, and face)
- Dysarthria (difficulty speaking)
- Dyskinesias (uncontrolled, involuntary movements)
- Dysphagia (problems swallowing)
- Dystonia (involuntary muscle contractions)
- Rhabdomyolysis
- Tremor
- Trismus

Other considerations

- Electrolyte and metabolic abnormalities
  - Hypocalcemia, hypomagnesemia, hypo- or hypernatremia, hypokalemia, and metabolic acidosis
- Elevated creatine kinase (CK): >1000 U/L
- Dehydration

- Leukocytosis: $> 11.0 \times 10^9$/L
- Treatment with dopamine antagonist (neuroleptic) medications within the previous 72 hours

DIFFERENTIAL DIAGNOSIS

Neurologic

- Acute cerebrovascular accident
- Acute hydrocephalus
- Malignant catatonia
- Meningitis or encephalitis
- Seizures

Cardiovascular

- Myocardial infarction
- Cardiogenic shock

Endocrine

- Pheochromocytoma
- Thyrotoxicosis

Musculoskeletal

- Malignant hyperthermia

Pharmacologic

- Anticholinergic overdose or poisoning
- Acute intoxication with cocaine, ecstasy, or methamphetamines
- Dopamine antagonist medications
- Serotonin syndrome

Other considerations

- Anaphylactic shock
- Delayed emergence from anesthesia
- Fever
- Heat stroke
- Hypovolemic shock
- Porphyria
- Septic shock
- Substance abuse withdrawal
- Tetanus

Diagnostic tests

- Electrolyte panel, calcium, magnesium, phosphorus
- Evaluate complete blood count for elevated white blood cell count

- Evaluate serum creatinine kinase, hepatic transaminases, lactate dehydrogenase, alkaline phosphatase
- Serum creatinine, blood urea nitrogen, and urine myoglobin
- Arterial blood gas
- Blood and urine toxicity screen
- Serum iron concentration
- Serum thyroid function studies (e.g., T3/T4/TSH)
- Point of care ultrasound (POCUS) of vena cava to evaluate fluid status
- Chest radiograph
- Electrocardiogram
- Computed tomography of the head

Suggested Readings

- Berman BD. Neuroleptic malignant syndrome: a review for neurohospitalists. *Neurohospitalist*. 2011;1(1):41-47.
- Simon LV, Hashmi MF, Callahan AL. Neuroleptic malignant syndrome. [Updated 2022 Apr 28]. In: *StatPearls* [Internet]. Treasure Island, FL: StatPearls Publishing; 2022. Available at: https://www.ncbi.nlm.nih.gov/books/NBK482282/.
- Oruch R, Pryme IF, Engelsen BA, Lund A. Neuroleptic malignant syndrome: an easily overlooked neurologic emergency. *Neuropsychiatr Dis Treat*. 2017;13:161-175. Published Jan 16, 2017.
- van Rensburg R, Decloedt EH. An approach to the pharmacotherapy of neuroleptic malignant syndrome. *Psychopharmacol Bull*. 2019;49(1):84-91.

CHAPTER 40   Emergency Cesarean Section

MANAGEMENT

PRIMARY ACTIONS:

- On admission of the patient to the labor and delivery unit:
  1. Obtain medical history, perform a physical examination, laboratory testing, and anesthesia consent
  2. Obtain large-bore peripheral IV access
     - Consider central venous access if peripheral IV access is difficult
  3. Evaluate the patient for difficult intubation risk factors
- Administer pharmacologic prophylaxis for gastric aspiration (see "Medications")
- Maintain left uterine displacement until delivery of the fetus
- Obtain type and screen
  - Obtain type and cross if vaginal bleeding is occurring
  - Consider activating the massive transfusion protocol if significant vaginal bleeding is evident (see "Medications")
  - Obtain fibrinogen and calcium values if significant hemorrhage with massive transfusion occurs
- Maintain effective communication with the surgical team and determine if neuraxial or general anesthesia is prudent, depending on maternal status and fetal condition
  - See Table 40-1 for signs and symptoms of indications for emergency cesarean delivery
- Neuraxial anesthesia should extend up to a T4 sensory level
  1. Epidural: administer local anesthetic, opioids, and/or adjuvants (e.g., nonopioid analgesics, epinephrine, sodium bicarbonate)
  2. Spinal: administer local anesthetic, opioids, and/or adjuvants (e.g., nonopioid analgesics, epinephrine)
- If general anesthesia is required, anesthesia induction should occur after surgery preparation is complete and the surgical staff is ready
  1. Perform a rapid sequence induction and intubation with cricoid pressure
  2. Consult the current American Society of Anesthesiologists' Difficult Airway Algorithm if necessary

SECONDARY ACTIONS:
- After delivery, administer uterotonic medication (see "Medications")
- Supportive measures, as necessary (see "Medications)
- Avoid lethal triad: acidosis, hypothermia, and coagulopathy
- Monitor acid-base, fluid, electrolyte balance, and quantitative blood loss
- If general anesthesia is used, extubate once the patient is awake and following commands, neuromuscular blockade is fully reversed, and the criteria for extubation have been met
- Consider transverse abdominal plane block for postoperative pain

MEDICATIONS:
- Aspiration prophylaxis
    - Nonparticulate antacid, sodium citrate 30 mL PO, immediately before surgery
    - Histamine H2 receptor antagonist, famotidine 20 mg IV, 40-90 minutes before induction
    - Gastrointestinal prokinetic, metoclopramide 10 mg IV, 30-60 minutes before induction
- Uterotonics
    - Oxytocin infusion 3-5 Unit IV bolus, 10 Unit/h infusion and/or,
    - Methylergonovine (Methergine) 0.2 mg IM every 2-4 hours as needed and/or,
    - Carboprost (Hemabate) 250 mcg IM every 15-90 minutes as needed, maximum total dose 2 mg and/or,
    - Misoprostol 600 to 1000 mcg as a single rectal or sublingual dose
- Vasopressor(s) to maintain MAP > 65 mm Hg:
    - Ephedrine 5-10 mg IV bolus and/or,
    - Phenylephrine 50-100 mcg IV bolus, 0.1-0.5 mcg/kg/min infusion and/or,
    - Epinephrine 10-100 mcg IV bolus, 0.1-0.5 mcg/kg/min infusion and/or,
    - Dopamine 5-20 mcg/kg/min IV infusion and/or,
    - Norepinephrine 5-10 mcg IV bolus, 0.1-0.5 mcg/kg/min infusion and/or,
    - Vasopressin 1-4 Unit IV bolus, 0.01-0.1 Units/min infusion
- Massive transfusion protocol is dependent on hospital protocol
    - Goal should be as close to a 1 PRBC – 1 FFP – 1 platelet ratio as possible
    - Consider administration of cryoprecipitate
    - Consider calcium supplementation (1 gram calcium gluconate IV over 10 minutes or 1 gram calcium chloride over 10 minutes administered through a central line)

Table 40-1 Signs and symptoms of indications for emergency cesarean delivery

	INDICATIONS	SIGNS AND SYMPTOMS
Maternal	Antepartum hemorrhage (e.g., placenta abruption)	• Abrupt onset vaginal bleeding (mild to severe) • Back or abdominal pain • Disseminated intravascular coagulation (DIC) • Fetal death • Fetal heart rate abnormalities • Firm, rigid, tender uterus • Hypotension • Preterm labor • Retroplacental hematoma viewed with obstetrical ultrasound
	Maternal distress (e.g., amniotic, pulmonary embolism)	• Acute respiratory failure (e.g., hypoxia, dyspnea) • DIC • Hemoptysis • Hypotension • Pleuritic chest pain • Seizures • Sudden-onset cardiorespiratory arrest
	Preeclampsia	• Abnormal liver function tests • Abnormal renal function tests • End-organ dysfunction • HELLP syndrome (Hemolysis, Elevated Liver enzymes, Low Platelets) • Hypertension, systolic blood pressure (BP) ≥ 160 or diastolic BP ≥ 110 • Proteinuria • Pulmonary edema • Thrombocytopenia • Visual symptoms (e.g., blurred vision, flashing lights/sparks)
Fetal	Fetal distress (e.g., abnormal, indeterminate fetal heart rate tracing)	• Absent baseline fetal heart rate variability • Recurrent late decelerations • Recurrent variable decelerations • Bradycardia • Sinusoidal pattern • Scalp stimulation that does not induce fetal heart rate acceleration

Continued

Table 40-1 Signs and symptoms of indications for emergency cesarean delivery—cont'd

	INDICATIONS	SIGNS AND SYMPTOMS
	Fetal malpresentation	• Breech • Brow • Compound • Face • Occiput posterior • Transverse lie
Other	Labor dystocia (e.g., protraction, arrest of labor)	• Protraction: cervical dilation ≥ 6 cm, with dilation < 1-2 cm over 2 h • Arrest: cervical dilation ≥ 6 cm, with no cervical change for ≥ 4 hours despite adequate contractions OR no cervical change for ≥ 6 h of oxytocin administration with inadequate contractions
	Placental disorder	• Placenta previa (placental tissue that extends over the internal cervical os) • Placenta accreta (placental villi attach to myometrium) • Placenta increta (placental villi penetrate the myometrium) • Placenta percreta (placental villi penetrate through myometrium to the uterine serosa or adjacent organs)
	Umbilical cord prolapse	• Overt: the umbilical cord moves ahead of the fetal presenting part and into the cervical canal, vagina, or externally • Occult: the umbilical cord moves adjacent to the fetal presenting part • Fetal bradycardia • Variable decelerations • Late decelerations • Palpation or visualization of the umbilical cord with examination

Table 40-1 Signs and symptoms of indications for emergency cesarean delivery—cont'd

INDICATIONS	SIGNS AND SYMPTOMS
Uterine rupture	• Severe abdominal pain (continues between contractions) • Abnormal contraction pattern • Abnormal fetal heart rate • Hematuria • Hypotension • Loss of fetal station • Tachycardia • Significant vaginal bleeding

PHYSIOLOGY AND PATHOPHYSIOLOGY

In the United States, approximately 30% of all births are performed by cesarean delivery. Anesthesia for emergency cesarean delivery focuses on ensuring the safety of the parturient and fetus/neonate. The choice of the anesthesia technique for cesarean delivery depends on the surgical urgency, which is determined by maternal status and fetal condition. Therefore, high-quality communication between the anesthesia provider, obstetrician, and nursing staff is essential.

An anesthesia consultation should be performed on the patient's admission to obtain a thorough medical history, physical examination, laboratory testing, and anesthesia consent. Several other factors will influence the choice of the anesthetic technique, such as a suboptimal coagulation status and/or difficult airway risk factors (e.g., increased body mass index, Mallampati score III or IV, small hyoid-to-mentum distance, limited jaw protrusion, limited mouth opening, cervical spine limitations). Pharmacological prophylaxis for gastric aspiration is prudent before anesthesia, given the anatomical and physiological changes associated with pregnancy.

If general anesthesia is planned, rapid sequence induction and intubation with cricoid pressure should be performed after adequate preoxygenation. Once endotracheal tube placement is confirmed, the surgical incision can be made. A minimum alveolar concentration (MAC) of inhalation anesthesia should be based on the patient's hemodynamic status. A lower MAC value (≤ 1) may be used to minimize intraoperative awareness while maintaining uterine tone after delivery. However, critically low blood pressure may necessitate a decreased MAC value.

The time between the surgical incision and delivery should be less than 3 minutes. An interval greater than 3 minutes is associated with neonatal depression and acidosis. Extubation is performed once the patient is awake and following commands. Neuromuscular blockade should be fully reversed, and the criteria for extubation have been met. Last, see Table 40-2 for Enhanced Recovery After Cesarean delivery recommendations.

SIGNS AND SYMPTOMS

See Table 40-1 for signs and symptoms of indications for emergency cesarean delivery.

DIFFERENTIAL DIAGNOSIS

Indications for emergency cesarean delivery

- Antepartum hemorrhage
- Fetal distress
- Fetal malpresentation
- Labor dystocia
- Maternal distress
- Placental disorder
- Preeclampsia

Table 40-2 Enhanced recovery after cesarean (ERAC) delivery recommendation

PHASE OF ANESTHESIA CARE	RECOMMENDATION
Preoperative	• Minimize fasting, clear liquids up to 2 h before surgery • Consider preoperative oral carbohydrate loading
Intraoperative	• Use of neuraxial anesthesia and intrathecal opioid (low dose) • Multimodal IV/IM analgesia • Antibiotic medication prophylaxis • Nausea and vomiting prophylaxis • Maintain normothermia (e.g., forced-air convective warming, warm IV fluids) • Maintain adequate IV hydration
Postoperative	• Early mother-neonate skin-to-skin contact

- Umbilical cord prolapse
- Uterine rupture

Diagnostic tests

- Complete blood count
- Fetal heart rate monitor (e.g., external, internal fetal scalp electrode)
- Tocodynamometry (e.g., external, internal/intrauterine pressure catheter)
- Obstetric ultrasound
- 24-hour protein urine collection
- Renal function tests
- Liver function tests
- Type and screen/crossmatch

Suggested Readings

- Clayton BA, Geisz-Everson MA, Wilbanks B. Thematic analysis of obstetric anesthesia cases from the AANA Foundation Closed Claims Database. *AANA J.* 2018;86(6):464-470.
- Mankikar MG, Sardesai SP, Ghodki PS. Ultrasound-guided transversus abdominis plane block for post-operative analgesia in patients undergoing caesarean section. *Indian J Anaesth.* 2016;60(4):253-257.
- Reale SC, Bauer ME, Klumpner TT, et al. Frequency and risk factors for difficult intubation in women undergoing general anesthesia for cesarean delivery: a multicenter retrospective cohort analysis. *Anesthesiology.* 2022;136(5):697-708. doi:10.1097/ALN.0000000000004173.
- Tubog TD, Ramsey VL, Filler L, Bramble RS. Minimum effective dose (ED50 and ED95) of intrathecal hyperbaric bupivacaine for cesarean delivery: a systematic review. *AANA J.* 2018;86(5):348-360.

CHAPTER 41   Obstetric Hemorrhage

MANAGEMENT

PRIMARY ACTIONS:

- Treat underlying pathological state
- Ensure surgical management/intervention
  1. Direct (manual) pressure to the wound or surgical site
  2. Use of topical hemostatic agents
  3. Surgical ligation or clamping of blood vessels
  4. Intrauterine tamponade, uterine compression suture, or hysterectomy
- Goal-directed crystalloid, colloid, factor concentrates, and blood product component therapy (e.g., administration based on clinical and laboratory assessment)
- Avoid lethal triad: acidosis, hypothermia, and coagulopathy
- If antepartum or intrapartum bleed, maintain left uterine displacement until delivery of fetus is viable

SECONDARY ACTIONS:

- Evaluate the patient for a potentially difficult intubation
- Supportive measures as necessary (see "Medications")
  1. Airway management and mechanical ventilation
  2. Invasive monitoring (e.g., arterial, central venous pressure)
  3. Monitor acid-base, fluid, and electrolyte balance
  4. Multiple large-bore peripheral IVs and/or central venous access
- Activate goal-directed massive transfusion protocol.
  - For example, 4 units packed red blood cells + 4 units fresh frozen plasma + 1 pooled platelet unit (e.g., equal to 4-6 individual units).
  - Consider adjunctive therapeutic agents (e.g., antifibrinolytics, fibrinogen concentrates)
- Consider autologous blood cell salvage and autotransfusion if there is a low risk of amniotic fluid present
- Type and cross
- Baseline arterial blood gas analysis
- Baseline hemoglobin, hematocrit, platelet, and electrolyte values
- Obtain fibrinogen level

MEDICATIONS:

- Uterotonics for postpartum hemorrhage
  - Oxytocin infusion 3-5 Unit IV bolus, 10 Unit/h infusion and/or,
  - Methylergonovine (Methergine) 0.2 mg IM every 2-4 hours as needed and/or,
  - Carboprost (Hemabate) 250 mcg IM every 15-90 minutes as needed, maximum total dose 2 mg and/or,
  - Misoprostol 600 to 1000 mcg as a single rectal or sublingual dose

- Antifibrinolytics
  - Aminocaproic acid 4-5 grams IV loading dose given over 1 hour, then 1 gram/h infusion for 8 hours and/or,
  - Tranexamic acid 10-30 mg/kg IV given over 10-30 minutes
- Recombinant Factor VIIa 70 to 90 mcg/kg/dose IV, every 2-3 hours until hemostasis is achieved
  - Avoid in patients with a coagulopathy, hypothermia, or acidosis
- Vasopressor(s) to maintain MAP > 65 mm Hg:
  - Ephedrine 5-10 mg IV bolus and/or,
  - Phenylephrine 50-100 mcg IV bolus, 0.1-0.5 mcg/kg/min infusion and/or,
  - Epinephrine 10-100 mcg IV bolus, 0.1-0.5 mcg/kg/min infusion and/or,
  - Dopamine 5-20 mcg/kg/min IV infusion and/or,
  - Norepinephrine 5-10 mcg IV bolus, 0.1-0.5 mcg/kg/min infusion and/or,
  - Vasopressin 1-4 Unit IV bolus, 0.01-0.1 Units/min infusion

PHYSIOLOGY AND PATHOPHYSIOLOGY

Obstetric hemorrhage is a significant cause of maternal morbidity and mortality. It may occur during the antepartum, intrapartum, or postpartum period. Obstetric patients have an increased circulating blood volume. Therefore, signs and symptoms of hypovolemia (e.g., tachycardia, hypotension) may only occur when volume depletion is extreme. Performing an accurate (quantitative) blood loss assessment is essential, as is the initiation of treatment when clinically indicated.

Antepartum hemorrhage (APH) can occur from 20 weeks' gestation to the onset of labor. Intrapartum hemorrhage (IPH) can occur between the onset of labor and delivery. APH and IPH can be caused by:
(1) abnormal placental attachment (e.g., placenta previa, accreta, increta, percreta)
(2) uteroplacental separation (e.g., placental abruption)
(3) uterine rupture or trauma
(4) fallopian tube rupture (e.g., ectopic pregnancy)
(5) fetoplacental vessel rupture (e.g., vasa previa)
(6) lower genital tract lesions (e.g., cervicitis, vaginal varices)
(7) spontaneous abortion

Postpartum hemorrhage (PPH) can occur following delivery and for up to 6 weeks after delivery. Postpartum hemorrhage is a blood loss greater than 500 mL after vaginal delivery and greater than 1000 mL after cesarean delivery. Uterine atony is a frequent cause of PPH. It results from the failure of endogenous maternal uterotonics (e.g., oxytocin, prostaglandins) to stimulate effective contractions, which typically compress uterine blood vessels following delivery. Other causes of PPH include: (1) retained products of conception, (2) abnormal placental attachment, (3) uterine inversion, (4) coagulopathy, (5) gynecological lacerations and tears, or (6) uterine rupture.

SIGNS AND SYMPTOMS

Neurologic

- Acute onset nausea/vomiting
- Altered level or loss of consciousness

Respiratory

- Cyanosis
- Hypercarbia
- Hypoxia
- Pallor
- Respiratory arrest

Cardiovascular

- Cardiac arrest
- Delayed capillary refill
- Dysrhythmias
- Hypertension (early compensatory sign of hemorrhage)
- Hypotension (late sign associated with hemorrhage)
- Tachycardia

Renal

- Decreased urine output

Hematologic

- Abnormal laboratory studies:
    1. Altered coagulation studies
    2. Decreased hemoglobin and hematocrit values
    3. Low fibrinogen value
- Disseminated intravascular coagulation (DIC)
- Indications of DIC or coagulopathy (e.g., oozing from puncture sites, uncontrolled bleeding)

Other considerations

- Abdominal pain
- Estimated blood loss > 1000 mL
- Fetal bradycardia or decelerations
- Vaginal or perineal bleeding

DIFFERENTIAL DIAGNOSIS

Obstetric considerations

- Amniotic fluid embolism
- Antepartum and intrapartum hemorrhage:
  1. Ectopic pregnancy
  2. Lower genital tract lesions (e.g., cervicitis, vulvovaginal varices)
  3. Placental abruption
  4. Placenta previa
  5. Uterine rupture
  6. Vasa previa
- Postpartum hemorrhage:
  1. Placenta accreta, increta, or percreta
  2. Retained placenta
  3. Trauma to obstetric anatomy (e.g., cervix, vagina)
  4. Uterine atony
  5. Uterine inversion
- Preeclampsia
- Uterine trauma

Cardiovascular

- Aortocaval compression
- Embolus (amniotic fluid)
- Hemorrhage
- Hypotension
- Hypovolemia

Renal

- Acute renal failure

Hematologic

- Coagulopathy (e.g., DIC, preeclampsia, anticoagulants, preexisting bleeding disorders, dilutional thrombocytopenia)

Other considerations

- Hypocalcemia
- Hypothermia
- Shock

Diagnostic tests

- Arterial blood gas
- Complete blood count
- D-dimer
- Fibrinogen

- Functional hemodynamic monitoring (e.g., stroke volume variation, pulse pressure variation, Pleth variability index)
- Prothrombin time, activated partial thromboplastin time, activated clotting time
- Serum electrolyte test(s): sodium, potassium, calcium, magnesium
- Thromboelastogram
- Type and screen/crossmatch
- Ultrasound (abdominal, uteroplacental)

Suggested Readings

- American Society of Anesthesiologists Task Force on Perioperative Blood Management. Practice guidelines for perioperative blood management: an updated report by the American Society of Anesthesiologists Task Force on Perioperative Blood Management. *Anesthesiology.* 2015;122(2):241-275. doi:10.1097/ALN.0000000000000463.
- Clayton BA, Geisz-Everson MA, Wilbanks B. Thematic analysis of obstetric anesthesia cases from the AANA Foundation Closed Claims Database. *AANA J.* 2018;86(6):464-470.
- Elisha S. Intraoperative maternal hemorrhage caused by uterine rupture. In: Elisha S, ed. *Case Studies in Nurse Anesthesia.* St. Louis, MO: Elsevier; 2022:261-266.
- Ranalli LJ, Taylor GA. Obstetric anesthesia. In: Elisha S, Heiner JS, Nagelhout JJ, eds. *Nurse Anesthesia.* 7th ed. St. Louis: Elsevier; 2023:1176-1206.

CHAPTER 42 Preeclampsia and Eclampsia

MANAGEMENT

PRIMARY ACTIONS:

- Definitive treatment is delivery of the fetus and placenta
- Maintain systolic blood pressure $<$ 160 mm Hg and diastolic blood pressure $<$ 110 mm Hg (see "Medications")
- Seizure prophylaxis and treatment (see "Medications")
- Goal-directed crystalloid, colloid, factor concentrates, and blood product component therapy (e.g., administration based on clinical and laboratory assessment)

SECONDARY ACTIONS:

- Monitor for HELLP syndrome (hemolysis, elevated liver enzymes, and low platelets)
- Assess coagulation status before neuraxial anesthesia (see "Diagnostic Tests")
- Supportive measures, as necessary (see "Medications")
  1. Airway management and mechanical ventilation
  2. Invasive monitoring (e.g., arterial, central venous catheter)
  3. Monitor acid-base, fluid, and electrolyte balance
  4. Multiple large-bore peripheral IVs or central venous access

MEDICATIONS:

- Antihypertensives
  - Nifedipine 30 mg PO and/or,
  - Labetalol 10-20 mg IV bolus over 1-2 minutes and/or,
  - Hydralazine 2.5-5 mg IV bolus every 10-15 minutes, up to 20 mg total dose and/or,
  - Methyldopa 250 mg PO every 8-12 hours
- Seizure Prophylaxis caused by eclampsia
  - Magnesium sulfate 4-6 grams IV loading dose over 15-30 minutes, followed by 1-2 g/h infusion for at least 24 hours after delivery
- Treatment of seizures caused by eclampsia
  - Magnesium sulfate 2-4 grams IV bolus over $\geq$ 5 minutes or
  - Midazolam 0.2 mg/kg IV bolus or
  - Lorazepam 4 mg IV bolus

PHYSIOLOGY AND PATHOPHYSIOLOGY

Preeclampsia is a condition that occurs during pregnancy and affects most organ systems. It is the third leading cause of maternal mortality. The disease can develop into severe preeclampsia and even eclampsia. Patient symptoms can include extreme hypertension, coagulopathy, pulmonary edema, renal dysfunction, liver dysfunction, myocardial infarction, cerebral edema, seizures (this indicates eclampsia), and intracranial hemorrhage.

The pathogenesis of preeclampsia is not entirely understood. However, the disease is associated with endothelial dysfunction. The high-resistance, low-perfusion placental circulation leads to oxidative stress. An imbalance of proangiogenic and antiangiogenic growth factors results in:

1. Platelet activation and consumption resulting in thrombocytopenia
2. Increased renal glomerular permeability causing proteinuria
3. Decreased production of vascular vasodilating substances
4. Increased vascular permeability
5. Increased sensitivity to endogenous vasoconstrictors such as norepinephrine and angiotensin

Risk factors for developing preeclampsia are numerous and include maternal obstetric factors, comorbid conditions (e.g., primary hypertension), genetics, lifestyle, and a history of preeclampsia. The progression of the disease is variable and may be severe when initially diagnosed. Without warning, preeclampsia may rapidly progress from mild to severe and finally to eclampsia.

SIGNS AND SYMPTOMS

Mild preeclampsia

- Hypertension (SBP > 140 mm Hg or DBP > 90 mm Hg)
- Proteinuria (> 300 mg per 24 hours)
- Edema/weight gain

Severe preeclampsia

- Hypertension (SBP > 160-180 mm Hg or DBP > 110 mm Hg)
- Severe proteinuria (> 5 g per 24 hours)
- Oliguria (< 500 mL/24 hours)
- Neurologic symptoms (e.g., headache, vision disturbances)
- Epigastric/right upper quadrant pain
- Intravascular fluid volume deficit
- Pulmonary edema

- HELLP syndrome:
  1. Hemolysis
  2. Elevated liver enzymes
  3. Low platelet count (thrombocytopenia)
- Renal dysfunction

Eclampsia

- New onset of grand mal seizures

Other possible signs and symptoms

- Fetal distress
- Intrauterine growth retardation
- Nausea and vomiting
- Oligohydramnios
- Paresthesias
- Pharyngolaryngeal edema

DIFFERENTIAL DIAGNOSIS

Neurologic

- Increased intracranial pressure (e.g., cerebral edema, intracranial mass)
- Intracranial aneurysm or hemorrhage
- Migraine headache
- Stroke
- Underlying seizure disorder

Cardiovascular

- Gestational hypertension
- Hypertension

Renal

- Acute renal failure
- Nephrotic syndrome
- Renal dysfunction

Endocrine

- Pheochromocytoma
- Thyroid storm

Hematologic

- Coagulopathy
- Disseminated intravascular coagulation
- Hemolytic anemia
- Thrombocytopenia

Gastrointestinal

- Gallbladder disease
- Pancreatic disease

Pharmacologic

- Local anesthetic toxicity (eclampsia and seizures)
- Magnesium toxicity
- Sympathomimetic drug use (e.g., cocaine, methamphetamine)

Other

- Malignant hyperthermia

Diagnostic tests

- 24-hour protein urine collection
- Arterial blood gas
- Complete blood count
- D-dimer
- Echocardiogram (e.g., transthoracic, transesophageal)
- Fibrinogen level
- Functional hemodynamic monitoring (e.g., stroke volume variation, pulse pressure variation, Pleth variability index)
- Liver function tests
- Prothrombin time, activated partial thromboplastin time, activated clotting time
- Renal function tests
- Serum electrolyte test(s): sodium, potassium, calcium, magnesium
- Thromboelastogram
- Type and screen/crossmatch

Suggested Readings

- Cunningham C, Rivera J, Spence D. Severe preeclampsia, pulmonary edema, and peripartum cardiomyopathy in a primigravida patient. *AANA J.* 2011;79(3):249-255.
- Elisha S. Cesarean section. In: Elisha A, ed. *Case Studies in Nurse Anesthesia.* St. Louis: Elsevier; 2022:251-256.
- Ranalli LJ, Taylor GA. Obstetric anesthesia. In: Elisha S, Heiner JS, Nagelhout JJ, eds. *Nurse Anesthesia.* 7th ed. St. Louis: Elsevier; 2023:1176-1206.
- Russell R. Preeclampsia and the anaesthesiologist: current management. *Curr Opin Anaesthesiol.* 2020;33(3):305-310. doi:10.1097/ACO.0000000000000835.

CHAPTER 43   Anesthesia Machine Malfunction

MANAGEMENT

PRIMARY ACTIONS:

- Call for help
- Notify the surgeon and stop the procedure if necessary
- Systematically assess for complications beginning at the patient and moving toward the anesthesia machine
- Maintain adequate airway, breathing, and circulation
  1. If a malfunction is not determined immediately, connect the patient to backup ventilation equipment using an auxiliary oxygen flowmeter or oxygen cylinder and a self-inflating manual resuscitation bag
  2. Ensure adequate oxygen E-cylinder supply (see "Medications")
  3. Continue physiological monitoring via transport monitor or traditional means (e.g., sphygmomanometer, palpation of pulses, auscultation of breath sounds)
- For an anesthetized patient
  1. Ensure delivery of anesthesia via total intravenous anesthesia
  2. If an infusion pump is unavailable, use manual dosing (see "Medications")

SECONDARY ACTIONS:

- Obtain a backup anesthesia machine

MEDICATIONS:

- Oxygen E-cylinder supply in hours = (PSI O_2 × 0.3)/(O_2 L/min × 60)
- Manual dosing for propofol (this is approximately 100 mcg/kg/min for a 50-kg patient)
  1. Intermittent manual bolus 2.5 mL every 5 minutes
  2. Microdrip tubing (60 drops/mL) 1 drop every other second

PHYSIOLOGY AND PATHOPHYSIOLOGY

The functions of an anesthesia machine are to assist the anesthesia provider in oxygenation and ventilation of the patient, carbon dioxide absorption, inhaled anesthetic delivery, and the safe removal of waste anesthetic gases from the scavenging system. Advanced technology has contributed to the rapid development of modern anesthesia delivery systems. Many newer anesthesia workstations are complex (e.g., digital interfacing, internalized components, computer software) and require continual maintenance and system updates. Therefore, anesthesia providers must be vigilant and maintain a detailed understanding of the anesthesia delivery system to provide safe patient care.

Figure 43-1 illustrates the basic functional structure of the anesthesia delivery system and includes a gas delivery system, patient breathing system, and scavenging system for waste gases. Malfunction of the anesthesia delivery system can occur at any level of this functional structure (Table 43-1). The low-pressure circuit is the "vulnerable area" of the anesthesia machine. The low-pressure system is subject to breakage and leaks, it is located downstream from all safety features (except the oxygen analyzer), and inappropriate low-pressure circuit testing will not detect malfunctions in this area. Manual and automated checklists function to assess the integrity of the anesthesia delivery system. Anesthesia providers must perform preanesthesia checkout procedures before every anesthetic. Table 43-2 provides recommendations for preanesthesia checkout procedures.

SIGNS AND SYMPTOMS

Respiratory

- Absent, increased, decreased, or abnormal capnography tracing
- Barotrauma or volutrauma
- Decreased ability to provide positive pressure ventilation
- Desaturation
- Fraction of inspired oxygen less than 25%
- Hypercarbia
- Hypoxia
- Inappropriately high or low inspired and expired tidal volume
- Inappropriately high or low peak inspiratory pressure
- Inappropriately high or low positive end-expiratory pressure

Cardiovascular

- Dysrhythmias
- Hypertension or hypotension
- Tachycardia or bradycardia

Pharmacologic

- Inappropriate carrier gas composition (e.g., oxygen, air, nitrous oxide)
- Inappropriately high or low concentration of inspired or expired inhalation anesthetic

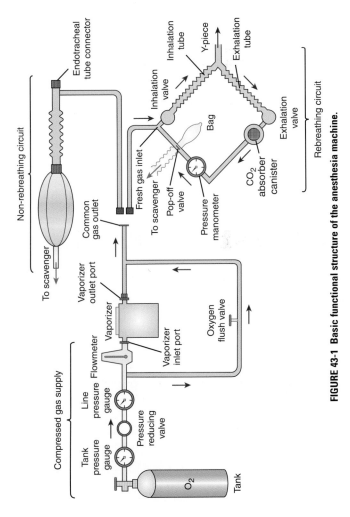

FIGURE 43-1 Basic functional structure of the anesthesia machine.

Table 43-1 Malfunctions associated with the anesthesia machine

DELIVERY SYSTEM	MALFUNCTION	SIGNS AND SYMPTOMS (S/S)
Gas delivery system	Gas supply source	• Fraction of inspired oxygen less than 25% • Inappropriate carrier gas composition (e.g., oxygen, air, nitrous oxide) • Inappropriate pressure of gas supply source • Low oxygen supply pressure alarm • Physiologic S/S could include hypoxemia, hypercarbia, and/or hypertension or hypotension
Patient breathing system	Anesthesia breathing circuit	• Absent or abnormal capnograph tracing • Barotrauma or volutrauma • Inappropriate peak inspiratory pressure • Physiologic S/S could include dysrhythmias, heart rate problems (e.g., bradycardia or tachycardia), and/or hypoxemia • Visual, auditory, and/or olfactory detection of an anesthetic gas leak
	Unidirectional valves	• Absent or abnormal capnography tracing • Barotrauma or volutrauma • Decreased ability to provide positive pressure ventilation • Inappropriate inspired and expired tidal volume • Inappropriate peak inspiratory pressure • Inappropriate positive end-expiratory pressure (PEEP) • Visual detection of unidirectional valve failure
	Vaporizer	• Intraoperative awareness or recall • Inappropriate concentration of inspired or expired inhalation anesthetic • Patient movement (if not paralyzed) • Physiologic S/S could include arrhythmias, heart rate problems (e.g., bradycardia or tachycardia), and/or hypertension or hypotension • Visual, auditory, and/or olfactory detection of an anesthetic gas leak

Table 43-1 Malfunctions associated with the anesthesia machine—cont'd

DELIVERY SYSTEM	MALFUNCTION	SIGNS AND SYMPTOMS (S/S)
Scavenging system	Scavenging system	• Inappropriate PEEP • Physiologic S/S could include hypoxemia • Visual, auditory, and/or olfactory detection of an anesthetic gas leak

Table 43-2 Recommendations for preanesthesia checkout procedures

1. Verify emergency ventilation equipment is available and functioning (e.g., oxygen cylinder and self-inflating manual ventilation device)
2. Verify patient suction is adequate to clear secretions/blood from the airway
3. Turn on the master switch to the anesthesia delivery system and confirm that electrical power is available
4. Check, calibrate, and set alarm limits for all physiological monitors
5. Check oxygen cylinder supply and verify that pressure is adequate on the emergency oxygen cylinder mounted on the anesthesia machine
6. Check central pipeline supplies and verify that the piped gas pressures are ≥ 50 PSI
7. Verify that vaporizers are filled and the filler ports are tightly closed
8. Perform a leak check of the low-pressure system and confirm no leaks in the gas supply between the flowmeters and the common gas outlet
   • Test flowmeters and verify the appropriate movement of the bobbins or floats
9. Adjust and check the scavenging system function
10. Calibrate the oxygen monitor and check the low oxygen alarm
11. Verify carbon dioxide absorbent is not exhausted
12. Perform pressure and leak check of the patient breathing system
13. Test patient ventilation system and unidirectional valves to verify that gas flows appropriately through the breathing circuit during both inhalation and exhalation
14. Document completion of checkout procedures
15. Confirm ventilator settings, evaluate the final readiness to deliver anesthesia care, and perform an anesthesia time out before induction of anesthesia

Other considerations

- Inappropriate pressure of gas supply source
- Intraoperative patient awareness or recall
- Low oxygen supply pressure alarm
- A malfunction during the preanesthesia checkout procedure
- Visual, auditory, and/or olfactory detection of an anesthetic gas leak
- See Table 43-1 for specific malfunctions

DIFFERENTIAL DIAGNOSIS

Respiratory

- Airway/operating room fire
- Anesthesia circuit disconnect
- Bronchospasm
- Endobronchial intubation
- Kinked ETT
- Mucus plug within endotracheal tube
- Pneumothorax
- Upper airway obstruction

Cardiovascular

- Cardiogenic shock
- Cardiac compressive shock
- Hypovolemic shock
- Pulmonary embolism

Other considerations

- Anaphylactic shock
- Carbon dioxide absorber depletion
- End-tidal CO_2 gas line disconnect
- Hypoxia actual or caused by mechanical malfunction/inaccuracy
- Malignant hyperthermia
- Serotonin syndrome
- Thyroid storm

Suggested Readings

- Brockwell RC, Dorsch J, Dorsch S, Eisenkraft J, Feldman J. *2008 ASA Recommendations for Pre Anesthesia Checkout.* Available at: https://www.asahq.org/standards-and-guidelines/2008-asa-recommendations-for-pre-anesthesia-checkout. Accessed June 8, 2023.
- Vinay B, Krishna KNG, Nitin M. Malfunction of the expiratory valve during spontaneous ventilation. *AANA J.* 2015; 83(6):400-402.
- Wren K, Condit MT. Anesthesia machine failure: a case study. *AANA J.* 2020;88(3):209-211.

CHAPTER 44   Electrical Power Failure

PRIMARY ACTIONS:

- Call for help
- Maintain adequate airway, breathing, and circulation
  1. If the anesthesia machine is not functioning, connect the patient to backup ventilation equipment using an auxiliary oxygen flowmeter or oxygen cylinder and a self-inflating manual resuscitation bag
  2. Ensure adequate oxygen E-cylinder supply (see "Medications")
  3. Continue physiological monitoring via transport monitor and physical assessment
- For an anesthetized patient
  1. Ensure the delivery of anesthesia via total intravenous anesthesia
  2. If an infusion pump is unavailable, manual administration of medications is warranted (see "Medications")
- Assess backup power and battery life of anesthesia machine and patient monitor

SECONDARY ACTIONS:

- Determine the estimated time for the return of power
- Discuss with the surgeon the need to continue surgery
- Gather emergency equipment (e.g., portable light source, airway equipment, monitoring equipment, emergency drugs)
- Assess the feasibility of transferring the patient to a location with electrical power

MEDICATIONS:

- Oxygen E-cylinder supply in hours = (PSI O_2 × 0.3)/(O_2 L/min × 60)
- Manual dosing for propofol (approximately 100 mcg/kg/min for 50-kg patient)
  1. Intermittent manual bolus 2.5 mL every 5 minutes
  2. Microdrip tubing (60 drops/mL) infusion 1 drop every other second

PHYSIOLOGY/PATHOPHYSIOLOGY

The electrical power to an operating room originates from the electrical company (or hospital emergency generator). The isolation transformer provides electrical power to standard and emergency electrical outlets throughout the operating rooms. Finally, electrical power is supplied to devices plugged into these outlets. Disruption of the electrical power circuit at any stage will cause partial or total electrical power failure in an operating room.

Immediate care for the patient during an electrical power failure includes (1) ensuring the adequacy of airway patency, breathing, and circulation, (2) providing appropriate patient monitoring, and (3) proper anesthesia management.

SIGNS AND SYMPTOMS

Loss of function of electrically powered equipment

Anesthesia equipment malfunction
- Advanced airway equipment (e.g., flexible intubating (fiberoptic) scope, video laryngoscope)
- Anesthesia machine (e.g., ventilator, desflurane vaporizer)
- Pharmaceutical dispensing device (e.g., Pyxis)
- Red indicator lights indicating imminent power loss
- Standard and invasive monitoring devices
  Operating room equipment malfunction
- Ambient and surgical lighting
- Cardiopulmonary bypass equipment
- Fluid and warming devices
- Operating room bed
- Surgical instruments (e.g., electrocautery, laparoscopy equipment)

DIFFERENTIAL DIAGNOSIS

- Anesthesia machine alarms
- Electrocution (e.g., microshock, macroshock)
- Extreme weather conditions
- Failure of electrical equipment
- Failure of electrical outlets
- Failure of emergency generator
- Failure of isolation transformer
- Internal or external hospital construction
- Natural disaster (e.g., fire, earthquake)
- Unplugged electrical equipment or power strip that is turned to the off position

Suggested Readings

- Holland EL, Hoaglan CD, Carlstead MA, et al. How do I prepare for OR power failure? *APSF Newsletter.* 2016;30(3):57-62.
- Vetter AG, Harman RJ, Stamper MJ, Titch JF, Vacchiano CA. Preparing for total power failure in the operating room. *AANA J.* 2019;87(4):291-297.
- Wren K, Condit MT. Anesthesia machine failure: a case study. *AANA J.* 2020;88(3):209-211.

CHAPTER 45 Delayed Emergence

MANAGEMENT

PRIMARY ACTIONS

- Maintain patent airway
- Ensure adequate oxygenation and ventilation
- Assess vital signs

SECONDARY ACTIONS

- Identify and manage cause(s)

PHARMACOLOGIC MANAGEMENT (SEE "MEDICATIONS"):

- Discontinue anesthetic medications (e.g., confirm inhalation agents and/or nitrous oxide are in the off position)
- Flumazenil for reversal of excessive/residual benzodiazepine administration
- Naloxone for reversal of excessive/residual opioid administration
- Sugammadex or anticholinesterase/anticholinergic for reversal of excessive/residual neuromuscular blocking agent
- Physostigmine treatment for central anticholinergic syndrome
- Intralipid treatment for local anesthetic systemic toxicity

METABOLIC AND ELECTROLYTE ABNORMALITY MANAGEMENT (SEE "MEDICATIONS"):

- Forced air warming and warmed fluid to treat hypothermia
- Dextrose 50% to treat hypoglycemia
- Regular insulin to treat hyperglycemia
- 3% hypertonic NaCl to treat hyponatremia
- Restore serum tonicity slowly with dextrose 5% or 0.45% NaCl solution to treat hypernatremia
- Calcium chloride or calcium gluconate for hypocalcemia
- Bisphosphonates for hypercalcemia
- Furosemide for hypermagnesemia
- Manage metabolic acidosis depending on cause (e.g., diabetic ketoacidosis, lactic acidosis, chronic kidney disease, diarrhea, toxin ingestion)

NEUROLOGICAL MANAGEMENT:

- Neurologic examination of pupils, cranial nerves, reflexes, and response to pain
- Neurosurgical consult
- Consider computed tomography and/or magnetic resonance imaging studies
- Intensive care monitoring with periodic neurologic assessment

MEDICATIONS

- Flumazenil 0.2 mg IV every minute up to 1 mg for reversal of benzodiazepines
- Naloxone 40 mcg IV every 2 minutes up to 400 mcg for reversal of opioids
- Sugammadex 1-4 mg/kg IV for reversal of neuromuscular blockade
- Physostigmine 0.5-2 mg IV over 2 minutes to treat central anticholinergic syndrome
- Intralipid 20% for local anesthetic systemic toxicity:
  - ≤70 kg: 1.5 mL/kg IV, followed by infusion at 0.25 mL/kg/minute IV
  - >70 kg: 100 mL IV, followed by infusion of 200-250 mL IV over 15-20 minutes
- Dextrose 50% 20-50 mL for hypoglycemia
- Regular insulin sliding scale for hyperglycemia
- 3% hypertonic NaCl at 1-2 mL/kg/h IV for hyponatremia
- 500-1000 mg 10% calcium gluconate IV over 5 minutes for hypocalcemia
- Furosemide 1 mg/kg IV for hypermagnesemia

PHYSIOLOGY AND PATHOPHYSIOLOGY

Delayed emergence occurs when a patient remains unconscious after anesthetic administration has been discontinued. Delayed emergence can most often be attributed to (1) the prolonged pharmacological actions of anesthetic agents, (2) metabolic or electrolyte abnormalities, (3) inadequate cerebral perfusion, (4) neurologic injury, and/or (5) the prolonged effects of other medications or toxins.

The most common cause of delayed emergence is the residual cerebral depressant effects of anesthetic medications. This may be the result of excessive drug administration, synergistic effects between central nervous system depressants, or alterations in drug pharmacokinetic/pharmacodynamic profiles based on genetic or environmental factors. Pharmacokinetic drug action can be altered by hepatic and/or renal disease. These conditions inhibit drug metabolism, decrease protein synthesis, and delay elimination. In contrast, pharmacodynamic drug actions are affected by extremes of age, hypothermia, comorbidities, or the simultaneous use of other central nervous system depressants (e.g., alcohol, substance misuse, or other sedatives). Delayed emergence can also occur from residual neuromuscular blockade. Residual neuromuscular blockade can prohibit effective ventilation, cerebral oxygenation, and patient awakening.

Delayed emergence may also be caused by metabolic and electrolyte aberrations such as hypoglycemia, severe hyperglycemia, acidosis, and hypothermia. A serum glucose of less than

50 mg/dL correlates with altered levels of consciousness. High serum glucose levels (e.g., > 600 mg/dL) may lead to diabetic ketoacidosis, dehydration, and coma. Acidosis can be caused by several factors and alters the homeostasis necessary for proper metabolism and elimination of medications. Hypothermia also affects drug metabolism causing prolonged effects. Sodium, calcium, and/or magnesium electrolyte abnormalities may affect central nervous, cardiovascular, respiratory, and musculoskeletal systems causing hypoventilation, altered circulation, hypoxemia, hypercarbia, acidosis, and delayed awakening.

Neurologic injury resulting in either a global or focal ischemic event can result in delayed emergence. Problems that may cause neurologic injury include cerebral trauma, cerebrovascular accident, embolic phenomena (e.g., thrombus, air, or fat), increased intracranial pressure, and hematoma formation (e.g., subdural or epidural). Cerebral hypoxia and/or an increased cerebral metabolic rate of oxygen consumption may also lead to neurologic damage and a decreased level of consciousness.

SIGNS AND SYMPTOMS

Neurologic

- Absent response to verbal or painful stimulus
- Altered level of consciousness
- Constricted/dilated/nonreactive pupils
- Disconjugate gaze
- History of cognitive (e.g., dementia) or psychiatric disorders
- Increased intracranial pressure > 15 mm Hg (Cushing triad: widening pulse pressure, bradycardia, irregular respirations)
- Loss of somatosensory and/or motor evoked potentials during tumor resection
- Seizures

Respiratory

- Hypercarbia
- Hypoxia
- Bradypnea or tachypnea

Cardiovascular

- Extreme hypertension
- Hypotension
- Dysrhythmias
- Myocardial ischemia/infarction

Musculoskeletal

- Decreased muscle tone or muscle flaccidity

Metabolic

- Decreased core temperature < 35 °C
- Blood glucose < 50 mg/dL or > 600 mg/dL
- Blood serum pH < 3.5

Electrolyte

- Hyponatremia, hypernatremia, hypocalcemia, hypercalcemia, hypermagnesemia

DIFFERENTIAL DIAGNOSIS

Neurologic

- Central anticholinergic syndrome
- Cerebral vascular accident
- Hydrocephalus
- Hypoperfusion (e.g., hypoxia, emboli, thrombus, shock)
- Increased intracranial pressure (e.g., cerebral trauma, subdural/epidural hematoma)
- Neurological surgery (e.g., tumor excision)
- Postoperative cognitive dysfunction
- Dementia
- Seizure (e.g., postictal state)

Respiratory

- Airway obstruction
- Atelectasis
- Bronchospasm
- Hypercarbia
- Hypoxia

Cardiovascular

- Hypotension
- Myocardial ischemia/infarction

Renal

- Acute or chronic renal dysfunction with decreased drug clearance

Hepatic

- Hepatic disease causing decreased drug metabolism

Endocrine

- Hypothyroidism
- Adrenal insufficiency

Musculoskeletal

- Neuromuscular disorders (e.g., myasthenia gravis, multiple sclerosis, Guillain-Barre syndrome)

Pharmacologic

- Medication error
- Prolonged effect of medications:
  1. Opioids
  2. Muscle relaxants
  3. Inhalation anesthetics
  4. Nitrous oxide
  5. Benzodiazepines
  6. Anesthesia induction agents
  7. Local anesthetic toxicity
  8. Anticholinergics (e.g., atropine, scopolamine)
  9. Illicit depressant drugs (e.g., cannabis, heroin)
  10. Alcohol intoxication

Other considerations

- Electrolyte abnormalities:
  1. Hyponatremia or hypernatremia
  2. Hypocalcemia or hypercalcemia
  3. Hypermagnesemia
- Hyperglycemia, severe
- Hypoglycemia
- Hypothermia
- Pseudocholinesterase deficiency
- Shock states
- Traumatic injury

Diagnostic tests

- Arterial blood gas
- Electrocardiogram
- Echocardiogram (for suspected cardiac cause)
- Electrolytes (specifically sodium, calcium, and magnesium)
- Renal and hepatic serum values
- Computed tomography or magnetic resonance imaging scans of the brain

Suggested Readings

- Cascella M, Bimonte S, Di Napoli R. Delayed emergence from anesthesia: what we know and how we act. *Local Reg Anesth.* 2020;13:195-206.
- Lee JJ, Kilonzo K, Nistico A, Yeates K. Management of hyponatremia. *CMAJ.* 2014;186(8):E281-E286.
- Odom-Foreren J, Brady JM. Postanesthesia recovery. In: Elisha S, Heiner JS, Nagelhout JJ, eds. *Nurse Anesthesia.* 7th ed. St. Louis: Elsevier; 2023:1282-1283.
- Thomas E, Martin F, Pollard B. Delayed recovery of consciousness after general anaesthesia. *BJA Educ.* 2020;20(5):173-179.

CHAPTER 46   Hypothermia

MANAGEMENT

PRIMARY ACTIONS:

- Treat underlying pathological state
- Provide 100% oxygen
- Decrease distributive heat loss by using forced-air convective warming a half-hour before induction
- Use active rewarming strategies: forced-air convective warming, warmed intravenous fluids, and warmed irrigation fluids
- Use passive rewarming strategies: cover the patient's head, cover the patient with warm surgical gown/blankets, provide a heat and moisture exchanger on the endotracheal tube or laryngeal mask airway to limit exhaled heat loss, and increase room temperature

SECONDARY ACTIONS:

- Treat shivering (see "Medications")
- Monitor acid-base, fluid, and electrolyte balance
- Avoid excessive warming and hyperthermia

MEDICATIONS:

- Antishivering
  - Meperidine 0.35-0.5 mg/kg IV
  - Tramadol 0.25-0.5 mg/kg IV
  - Clonidine 0.5-1 mcg/kg IV
  - Dexmedetomidine 0.3-0.5 mcg/kg IV

PHYSIOLOGY/PATHOPHYSIOLOGY

The hypothalamus maintains temperature regulation of the human body to a core temperature of 37 °C ($\pm$ 0.5 °C). The hypothalamus: (1) receives sensory input from central and peripheral thermoreceptors; (2) promotes conscious thermoregulatory behavior; and (3) initiates autonomic responses of thermoregulation based on the core body temperature. Autonomic responses to hypothermia include vasoconstriction, nonshivering thermogenesis, and shivering thermogenesis.

Perioperative hypothermia is a core body temperature of less than 36°C. Conditions such as (1) decreased basal metabolic rate and heat production, (2) decreased perfusion to central and peripheral tissues, and (3) altered hypothalamic temperature regulation can predispose patients to hypothermic states. Perioperative hypothermia commonly occurs during two intraoperative phases: redistribution heat loss and continuous heat loss. Redistribution heat loss occurs after general and/or neuraxial anesthesia induction. Peripheral vasodilation causes heat transfer from the core to peripheral tissues. This transfer of heat can significantly decrease the core temperature by as much as 1° to 1.6°C. Mechanisms promoting continuous heat loss include radiation, convection, evaporation, and conduction.

SIGNS AND SYMPTOMS

Neurologic
• Altered level of consciousness

Respiratory
• Hypoxemia
• Ventilation/perfusion mismatch

Cardiovascular
• Cardiac dysfunction
• Dysrhythmias
• Myocardial infarction
• Peripheral vasoconstriction and/or piloerection

Hematologic
• Coagulopathy

Musculoskeletal
• Shivering

Pharmacologic
• Prolonged drug metabolism

Other Considerations
• Core body temperature less than 36°C
• Continuous heat loss
  1. Radiation: Transfer of body heat to a cool environment
  2. Convection: Exposure of tissues to circulating cool air or liquid, such as the infusion of cold intravenous fluids and blood products
  3. Evaporation: Cold and unhumidified inspired gases and/or exposed viscera
  4. Conduction: Direct contact with cold operating room equipment such as operating room table

DIFFERENTIAL DIAGNOSIS

Neurologic

- Depressed hypothalamic function
  1. Anesthetic medications
  2. Extremes of age
  3. Intracranial neoplasm
  4. Neurovascular pathology
  5. Traumatic brain injury
- Seizure

Cardiovascular

- Shock states

Endocrine

- Myxedema coma
- Panhypopituitarism

Other Considerations

- Exposure to extreme cold temperatures
- Inaccurate monitoring
- Permissive hypothermia
  1. Cardiopulmonary bypass
  2. Deep hypothermic circulatory arrest
  3. Neurosurgical hypothermic techniques
- Redistribution heat loss
  1. Inadequate forced-air warming, half-hour before induction
- Vascular insufficiency at the monitoring site

Suggested Reading

- Chakrabarti D, Kamath S, Deepti BS, Masapu D. Simple cost-effective alternative to fluid and blood warming system to prevent intraoperative hypothermia. *AANA J*. 2017;85(1):28-30.
- Roberson MC, Dieckmann LS, Rodriguez RE, Austin PN. A review of the evidence for active preoperative warming of adults undergoing general anesthesia. *AANA J*. 2013;81(5):351-356.
- Steelman VM, Schaapveld AG, Perkhounkova Y, Reeve JL, Herring JP. Conductive skin warming and hypothermia: an observational study. *AANA J*. 2017;85(6):461-468.

CHAPTER 47 Transurethral Resection of the Prostate (TURP) Syndrome

MANAGEMENT

PRIMARY ACTIONS

- Stop the infusion of irrigating fluid to the surgical site
- Administer high-flow oxygen by face mask when appropriate
- Maintain airway patency and adequacy of breathing/circulation
- Limit intravenous fluid administration
- Obtain hemoglobin, hematocrit, and serum electrolytes to assess for anemia and hyponatremia
- Administer an anticonvulsant to increase the seizure threshold and inhibit seizure activity
  1. benzodiazepine (e.g., midazolam)
  2. propofol (caution with administration if severe hypotension exists)

SECONDARY ACTIONS

- Redraw serum electrolytes every 20 minutes to assess for resolving hyponatremia
- Consider IV diuretic with congestive heart failure and/or severe hyponatremia (see "Medications")
- Consider IV administration of 3% hypertonic saline for serum sodium < 120 mEq/L (see "Medications")
  - Caution: Central pontine myelinolysis occurs with a 3% hypertonic infusion rate > 100 mL/h and/or a correction rate > 8 mEq/L in any 24-hour period
- Perform ACLS or PALS per American Heart Association protocol

MEDICATIONS

- Furosemide 20-40 mg IV bolus
- 3% hypertonic sodium chloride IV infusion rate of < 100 mL/h

PHYSIOLOGY AND PATHOPHYSIOLOGY

During specific endoscopic procedures (e.g., TURP, hysteroscopy) the instillation of fluids allows for bladder or uterine distention, irrigation, and improved surgical visualization. TURP syndrome occurs when an excessive volume of irrigating solution (sorbitol or glycine) is absorbed into the systemic circulation. The resulting intravascular hypervolemia causes circulatory overload and dilutes serum sodium and plasma proteins. These serum components diffuse out of the intravascular space and into the interstitial space. The relative hyponatremia can cause mild, moderate, or severe neurologic and cardiac dysfunction (Table 47-1). Factors that influence the amount of irrigating fluid absorbed include:

1. Duration of the surgical resection (ideally < 60 minutes)
2. Hydrostatic pressure of the irrigating fluid (determined by the height of the irrigation fluid bags relative to the patient)
3. Peripheral venous pressure
4. Quantity of open venous sinuses

Treatment of hyponatremia, caused by TURP syndrome, includes decreasing intravascular volume, which decreases the intravascular pressure gradient and promotes mobilization of serum sodium and plasma proteins back into the intravascular space.

Table 47-1 Neurological and cardiac manifestations resulting from dilutional hyponatremia

SERUM SODIUM (mEq/L)	NEUROLOGIC MANIFESTATIONS	CARDIAC MANIFESTATIONS
120	• Dizziness • Headache • Nausea	• Hypotension • Decreased myocardial contractility • Initial widening of QRS complex
115	• Vomiting • Restlessness • Confusion • Somnolence	• Bradycardia • Widening QRS complex • Elevated ST-segment • Ventricular ectopy • T-wave inversion
110	• Loss of consciousness • Seizures • Respiratory arrest	• Ventricular tachycardia • Ventricular fibrillation • Asystole

SIGNS AND SYMPTOMS

• See Table 47-1: Neurologic and cardiac manifestations associated with dilutional hyponatremia

Respiratory

• Cough
• Shortness of breath
• Wheezes, crackles, or rales on auscultation

Cardiovascular

- Cardiac arrest
- Dysrhythmias
- Jugular vein distention
- Tachycardia

Other considerations

- Visual abnormalities (e.g., decreased visual acuity, blurred vision)

DIFFERENTIAL DIAGNOSIS

Neurologic

- Increased intracranial pressure (e.g., cerebral edema, intracranial mass)
- Primary seizure disorder
- Transient ischemic attack/cerebrovascular accident

Respiratory

- Acute gastric aspiration
- Acute pulmonary edema

Cardiovascular

- Congestive heart failure
- Hypervolemia
- Myocardial ischemia/infarction

Renal

- Acute renal failure

Endocrine

- Hypoadrenalism
- Hypoglycemia
- Hypothyroidism
- Syndrome of inappropriate antidiuretic hormone secretion

Pharmacologic

- Local anesthetic systemic toxicity

Other considerations

- Anemia
- Glycine toxicity

Diagnostic tests

- Chest X-ray
- Electrocardiogram
- Laboratory tests: hemoglobin/hematocrit, electrolytes

Suggested Readings

- Elisha S. Transurethral resection of the prostate. In: Elisha S, ed. *Case Studies in Nurse Anesthesia*. St. Louis: Elsevier; 2022:289-295.
- Morse CY. Renal anatomy, physiology, pathophysiology, and anesthesia management. In: Elisha S, Heiner JS, Nagelhout JJ, eds. *Nurse Anesthesia*. 7th ed. St. Louis: Elsevier; 2023:742-769.
- Seif NE, Shehab HA, Elbadawy AM. Prophylaxis versus treatment against transurethral resection of prostate syndrome: the role of hypertonic saline. *Anesth Essays Res*. 2020; 14(1):104-111.

INDEX

Note: Page numbers followed by f indicate figures, t indicate tables, and b indicate boxes.